KU-354-557

MANAGING CRISIS AND
CHANGE IN HEALTH CARE

MANAGING CRISIS AND CHANGE IN HEALTH CARE
The organizational response to HIV/AIDS

CHRIS BENNETT
EWAN FERLIE

Open University Press
Buckingham • Philadelphia

Open University Press
Celtic Court
22 Ballmoor
Buckingham
MK18 1XW

and

1900 Frost Road, Suite 101
Bristol, PA 19007, USA

First Published 1994

Copyright © Chris Bennett and Ewan Ferlie 1994

All rights reserved. Except for the quotation of short passages for the
purposes of criticism and review, no part of this publication may be
reproduced, stored in a retrieval system, or transmitted, in any form or
by any means, electronic, mechanical, photocopying, recording or
otherwise, without the prior written permission of the publisher or a
licence from the Copyright Licensing Agency Ltd. Details of such licences
(for reprographic reproduction) may be obtained from the Copyright
Licensing Agency Ltd of 90 Tottenham Court Road, London, W1P 9HE.

A catalogue record of this book is available from the British Library

ISBN 0 335 15787 4 (pbk)   0 335 15788 2 (hbk)

Library of Congress Cataloging-in-Publication Data
Bennett, Chris, 1943–
    Managing crisis and change in health management: the
organizational response to HIV/AIDS / Chris Bennett, Ewan Ferlie.
        p.   cm.
    Includes bibliographical references and index.
    ISBN 0–335–15788–2 (cloth)   ISBN 0–335–15787–4 (pbk.)
    1. AIDS (Disease)—Government policy—Great Britain. 2. National
Health Service (Great Britain) 3. Delivery of Health Care—
organization & administration—Great Britain. I. Ferlie, Ewan,
1956– . II. Title.
    [DNLM: 1. Acquired Immunodeficiency Syndrome. 2. National Health
Service (Great Britain) 3. State Medicine—Great Britain.
4. Delivery of Health Care—history—Great Britain. 5. Public
Policy—Great Britain. WD 308 B471m 1994]
RA644.A25B447 1994
362.1'969792'00941—dc20
DNLM/DLC
for Library of Congress   93–50137   CIP

Typeset by Graphicraft Typesetters Limited, Hong Kong
Printed in Great Britain by St Edmundsbury Press, Bury St Edmunds, Suffolk

Contents

Acknowledgements

We have benefited from the help and advice of many people in the research which formed the basis of this book. Without their generous help and cooperation we could not have made sense of the complexity of events and relationships involved in the development of services for HIV/AIDS. A number of our collaborators spent considerably more time in helping us to achieve a higher level of understanding than we could reasonably have requested. Of course any failing of data collection or of interpretation should be laid at our door rather than theirs.

Among this group we would particularly like to thank: Dr George Bath, Yasmin Batliwala, Dr Peter Bellamy, Dr Ian Blair, Josie Burch, Dr Deidre Cunningham, James Fishwick, Phil Garner, Dr Rod Griffiths, Dr Joyce Leeson, Tim Matthews, Tom Matthews, Dr Dick Mayon-White, Helen Rushworth, David Sloman, Louis Smidt, Carol Tinto, Cathy Walter and Barbara Young. They made us feel more like trusted colleagues than strangers during our lengthy time in their health authorities.

We are also grateful to a number of fundors for their support. While this manuscript has been written in thematic rather than case-study-based terms, it has been dependent for its database on earlier commissioned case study work. We would particularly like to thank: Dr Lisa Catan, Dr Doreen Rothman and Dr Elizabeth Wilson at the Research Management Division of the Department of Health, Michael Brown, Alan Davey, Linda Johnson-Laird and Tom Snee from the Department of Health AIDS Unit, Helen George, Dr Mike George and Liz Jones at the Welsh Office, Dr Maryan

Pye from the Health Education Authority, Louis Smidt from the then Bloomsbury DHA and Andy Black from the then Parkside DHA.

We are grateful for stimulating conversations with academic colleagues, in particular Dr Virginia Berridge, Stephen Cranfield, Dr Charlotte Feinmann, Dr Ray Fitzpatrick and Dr Phil Strong.

We were encouraged greatly by our immediate colleagues at the Centre for Corporate Strategy and Change. In particular, we would want to acknowledge the enormous debt owed to our Director, Professor Andrew Pettigrew, both for his overall intellectual guidance and also his very practical help in undertaking personally some fieldwork for the project. We would also like to acknowledge the help and patience of the secretarial staff in the CCSC, Gill Drakeley and Ann Jackson.

This is a truly team-based and jointly authored manuscript: the ordering of the authors is alphabetical and not hierarchical. Indeed, as the book indicates, hierarchies may be giving way to networks.

Abbreviations

ACMD	Advisory Council for the Misuse of Drugs
AIDS	acquired immunodeficiency syndrome
AZT	azidothymidine (zidovudine)
BMA	British Medical Association
DHA	district health authority
GLF	gay liberation front
GP	general practitioner
HIV	human immunodeficiency virus
HTLV	human T-cell lymphoma virus
ICI	Imperial Chemical Industries
NHS	National Health Service
RCN	Royal College of Nursing
SMO	social movement organization
THT	Terrence Higgins Trust

CHAPTER
1

Crisis and change – the organizational response to HIV/AIDS

Introduction and rationale

The emergence of the HIV/AIDS epidemic in the 1980s was one of the most important – yet unheralded – developments in British health and social care during that decade. It presented a major challenge to existing service systems but it also offered an opportunity to respond to a new issue in new ways.

The first American reports of AIDS cases did not come through until 1981, and yet by late 1986 a full scale national 'crisis' was being constructed around the issue. However, by the late 1980s, the HIV/AIDS issue was slipping down the national agenda, while at the same time the number of reported AIDS cases continued to rise. As the epidemic became more of a social problem, paradoxically, it became less of a focus for policy attention. By the early 1990s, an infrastructure of services had been built up nearly everywhere, but especially in high prevalence, usually inner-city, settings.

The epidemic has had enormous implications for the communities most tragically affected, and indeed for society as a whole, and to conceive it in terms of a disaster is fully justified. Despite this, however, there have been some positive consequences; stimulation of much research and development activity from the medical professions, and new recognition of the importance of taking a collaborative approach to patient care as a result of pressure for change from grass roots voluntary organizations. Mann and Carballo (1989) indeed strike a note of real optimism in their comment that:

> One of the achievements of our era has nevertheless been the birth of global solidarity – imperfect, struggling, yet nevertheless real – in the creation of the United Nations, in the concern about nuclear war and, more recently, in the growing world-wide resolve to protect the common environment and prevent AIDS.

Some, however, would undoubtedly question that resolve, seeing such optimism as unjustified when world politicians, despite their oratory, 'know that the necessary funding will not be forthcoming' (FitzSimons 1993).

Our interest lies in one relatively small-scale – yet we would contend under investigated – aspect of this much bigger picture, namely developing an understanding of the organizational and managerial response to the HIV/AIDS epidemic. Britain in the 1980s was also characterized by a growing interest in the management process, and the empowerment of management as a social grouping under the doctrine of 'management must manage' was evident. In the NHS, old-style administration was replaced by new-style general management in the mid-1980s, and although these were often the same people, there were often significant developments in role (Pettigrew et al. 1992). For the newly appointed general managers, HIV/AIDS was perhaps the first 'new' issue to come along and to make a claim on their attention, though as we shall see, in the end much of the managerial response to the epidemic has come from the medical profession. Other organizations – notably voluntary organizations and social services departments – must also be seen as key components of the response, which went well beyond health care organizations.

The two fundamental concepts in our formulation of the problem are 'issue' and 'organization'. First, we conceive of HIV/AIDS as a public policy 'issue'. It is, of course, only one of the issues claiming the time, attention and resources of some of the complex multi-issue organizations involved (the NHS and social services departments), whilst at the same time being the only focus for some newly created voluntary organizations. We see it as being characterized by an issue 'lifecycle', moving from rapid early growth (1982–86), full-scale crisis (1986–87) and then slow decline as a public issue (1987–93), although not as a social problem. Organizations involved in the HIV/AIDS field may reflect a similar move from fluidity to routine. Chapters 2 and 3 provide a more detailed anatomy of HIV/AIDS as a public policy issue, and outline some of the key settings in which service activity was concentrated.

Second, we focus on patterns of organizational behaviour apparent in response to this new issue. Lead questions include: 'How have new services been developed and organized?' 'What is the nature of the management processes that have been instituted to respond to the epidemic?' 'Who has led this process of innovation?' It should be re-emphasized that we define the term 'organization' broadly so as to encompass a wide variety of sources of collective action, including both the 'official' health and social care systems and the 'alternative' voluntary sector. Indeed, the differences, and at times conflict, between these two very different types of organization form a major theme in the book.

There is now some work comparing the response to HIV/AIDS at a national level (Fox et al. 1989). There is also some American work examining the response in different localities, both from the perspective of higher journalism (Shilts 1987) and from more academic authors (Thomas and Fox 1989; Perrow and Guillen 1990). There is an important interest from contemporary historians (Berridge and Strong 1993), which reminds us of the historical analogies and templates (tuberculosis, syphilis, hepatitis). Amid apparently all-pervasive change, there were also subtle signs of continuity.

However, there remains a serious dearth of British studies examining the issues from a perspective informed by organization theory of local patterns of service evolution and of decision making (while Pye et al. (1989) tackle this area, their approach is highly empiricist). It is at the level of the individual hospital, health authority, social care or voluntary organization that many of the interesting questions about patterns of service innovation arise. The focus in this book is therefore very much on how such patterns of local organizational processes developed over time, and we hope it will make a distinctive contribution to the literature within the field of HIV/AIDS.

In addition, we would argue that the analysis of organizational change in relation to a specific issue and within particular settings has the potential not only to contribute to an understanding of the field, and therefore assist those involved in it, but to shed new light on generic influences on change that are relevant in other, quite different, contexts. The important themes in this book are all current subjects of management enquiry in both the public and private sectors. We believe much that is new can be derived from the analysis of change processes in relation to HIV/AIDS.

Approach to methodology

Research methods

The basic approach has been that of the longitudinal and processual comparative case study. As we have argued:

In summary, despite the substantial literature which now exists on change in health care organizations, we believe that there is a need for more research which is processual (an emphasis on action as well as structure); comparative (a range of studies of local health care agencies); pluralist (describe and analyse the often competing versions of reality seen by actors in change processes); and historical (take into account the historical evolution of ideas and actions for change as well as the constraints within which decision makers operate.

(Pettigrew et al. 1988: 314)

The case study has been a methodology as much abused as used, but case studies at their best can capture the richness of context and process in a way that is distinctively different, and may for some purposes be more useful than data collected using more quantitative methods and larger samples (Yin 1989). However, it is important to be clear about method. The approach adopted here has allowed for the retrospective analysis of change, as well as considerable real-time analysis. The antecedent conditions and the chronology of change are considered important historical elements, as the past may play a substantial part in shaping the characteristics of the present.

Our choice of design has been to conduct intensive analyses of a relatively few cases, rather than a more superficial analysis of a larger number. There is nothing intrinsically meritorious in having a large sample and, given the complexity of both the issue and the host organizations, superficial analyses could have at best provided only limited information and at worst might have been profoundly misleading. In fact Miller and Friesen (1982) have argued that if the material collected is valuable, even a single case study can sometimes be adequate.

The database for this work has been accumulated since 1987. It comprises six major case studies of English health authorities' responses to HIV/AIDS in and outside London, one case study in Scotland and two smaller English studies focusing on particular aspects of the response. In addition we have carried out extensive evaluation and dissemination work in this field for the Department of Health and the Welsh Office. In the course of this work we have carried out more than 600 formal interviews, most of which were tape-recorded, analysed a mass of archival material and attended numerous meetings at all levels of the organizations studied.

Respondents came from different functional groupings, different hierarchical levels and from organizations outside as well as inside the NHS (such as social services and voluntary organizations). Selection from such a wide pool of potential respondents was necessitated by the nature of the issue, but also increased the range of perspectives on the change process.

There was an extensive programme of feedback to the case study sites, and to 27 other authorities, as part of dissemination workshops funded by the Department of Health. This provided an excellent opportunity to validate our findings and also provided new data from a wider selection of localities.

Dialogue between theory and data

Our proposition in the development of case study work is that there should be dialogue between theory and data. Our plea for a shift of focus towards the micropolitics of the organization (and indeed of the interorganizational network) should not pave the way to endless and purely descriptive case studies. That would be to collude with the atheoretical empiricism of much British social science.

There needs to be the generation of a grounded theory, which can link theory and data (Glaser and Strauss 1967). Rudimentary concepts emerge out of early case data (e.g. crisis management, product champions, social movements). We then turn to theory to refine these concepts, which can then be reapplied to the case study data. In this fashion, it becomes easier to generalize from the data and to connect with wider bodies of social scientific literature.

In order to generate grounded theory, it is helpful to undertake comparative case study work where there is likely to be variability in outcomes (in the organizational rather than the clinical sense) between the sites in the sample. We can then begin to ask such questions as: 'Why was *this* the organizational outcome in site A, but *that* the organizational outcome in site B?' This approach was found to be useful in an earlier analysis of variation in the rate and pace of strategic change between district health authorities (Pettigrew et al. 1992) in which a more general model was derived inductively from the cross-case data.

Our data are derived from a mix of high, medium and low prevalence areas. However, low prevalence areas were under-represented in the sample, as we tended to study places where much had happened. Hence one should be cautious in extrapolating from the sample to the population.

A longitudinal approach

Another methodological point relates to the importance of time. We need to employ a longitudinal approach if we are to understand the full career of the HIV/AIDS issue and also the importance of local antecedent traditions in shaping the response to this issue. This may call for the skills of the historian in the analysis of archival material, as well as the interviewing skills of the sociologist. Many of our case studies stretch back long before the decade in which HIV/AIDS has been an issue, being a mixture of retrospective and real-time analysis.

Ferlie (1992) considers the methodological question of the relationship between the perspectives of history and of organization theory. While some branches of organization theory (such as the contingency theoretic approach popular in the 1960s and 1970s) are indeed ahistorical, other methodologies are far more sensitive to the importance of history in shaping organizational power structures, attitudes and assumptions. Within management studies, Chandler's (1977) classic analysis essentially represents a business history of the rise of the modern corporation as an institutional form and of management as a social grouping.

In the 1980s, there has been, if anything, a growing move within organization theory towards more processual and historical perspectives (e.g. Pettigrew's (1985) study of strategic change processes within ICI). The lifecycle and organizational transitions approaches to the study of organizations indeed organize themselves explicitly around the passage of time.

At the same time, there is a continued influence of sociology on those branches of organization theory which are sympathetic to historically informed analysis. As a result, there is a greater emphasis on the building and testing of formal theoretical models than in many purely historical accounts, although the pluralist nature of reality is acknowledged and competing interpretations of the past presented. There are thus areas of overlap and continuity of interest between the disciplines. The potential for a fruitful dialogue between history and organization theory is now apparent.

Key organizational themes

Clearly the HIV/AIDS issue is of major societal importance in its own right, as will be explored in Chapter 2. However it may also be used as a tracer for themes apparent in the organizational literature. The chapter structure of this book has been devised so as to give the maximum space to addressing what we consider to be some of the most important and generic organizational and managerial themes arising from the HIV/AIDS issue. Accordingly, following two chapters devoted to some essential 'scene-setting', Chapters 4–8 consider:

- ideologically driven change;
- issue recognition;
- entrepreneurialism, coalition building and crisis management;
- working across organizational boundaries;
- processes of individual, group and organizational learning.

We do not suggest that the response to HIV/AIDS can be seen as 'typical', but rather represents the experience of management under conditions of high policy drama. Such conditions may, however, expose decision-making processes that would otherwise remain hidden. Turner (1957) was, for example, an early exponent of using social dramas to illuminate process. At a general level, therefore, we need to address the debate about the applicability of organization theory to public and voluntary sector settings.

Organization theory applied to public and voluntary sector settings

Our treatment of the themes of this book is both empirically based and theoretically grounded, usually within organization theory but sometimes more widely in social studies. We make no apology for this, and indeed would argue strongly that an explicit awareness of theory broadens empirically and practice-driven perspectives. In the 1980s, the pendulum swung too violently away from any long-term concern for the research and development base, and it is now important for management scholars to affirm the advantages of more academic values.

We attempt in this book to apply organization theory to the analysis of an issue that arose mainly in public and voluntary sector service delivery settings. There are aspects of the HIV/AIDS epidemic that affect private firms, often to do with human resource policy, but we do not consider these aspects here.

Surely it can be objected that an alien body of literature developed in a private sector context is being applied in quite a different setting. We agree that it is a mistake to trundle concepts and models mindlessly across sectoral divides as organizational context is so important. However, it is also important that the study of public and voluntary sector organizations should not be ghettoized and marginalized from developments in wider fields of organizational study.

Our first response to this critique is that organization theory has a long tradition of drawing on public and voluntary sector settings. It is not true that all concepts have been derived from work in private sector settings. For example, the study of an innovative medical school contributed to the formation of the organizational lifecycle perspective (Kimberly and Miles 1980). Hospitals have also provided research settings for contingency theorists (de Kervasdoue 1981), students of professionalized organizations (Bucher and Stelling, 1977) and the validity of the population ecology perspective has been tested within the field of voluntary social service organizations (Singh et al. 1986).

Our second point is that there may be some room for creative intersectoral learning. Concepts and models brought in from wider settings may broaden the way that we see things and, even if they are not to be transported literally, may at the very least start a conversation about how we may develop analytical perspectives. We use notions of 'crisis management' and of 'product champions' in later chapters to help explain unfolding organizational processes. Both of these concepts were in fact developed in private sector settings, but may have more general relevance.

In the 1980s, the hardnosed, performance measurement-based approach, or the 'new managerialism', became increasingly prevalent in many public service settings, characterized by: tighter line hierarchies, stronger forms of accountability upwards, a greater focus on value for money and the setting and monitoring of objectives. While Pollitt (1990) exaggerates the extent to which this was the only public management style evident in the 1980s, his central point is sound. Yet in the private sector (e.g. Moss Kanter 1989), the talk was increasingly of moving towards more flexible, creative and self-managing organizational forms.

HIV/AIDS is of interest in these terms because it represented a new issue for the public sector, but one where many of the approaches advocated by the 'new managerialism' were difficult to apply. No doubt there will be a process of normalization and of routinization as the lifecycle of the epidemic progresses. There was, however, in the early years, a major need for creativity, inventiveness and flexibility. The level of uncertainty was such that it was difficult to set and monitor unambiguous objectives, but rather it was important to learn how best to respond. Leadership came less from general managers and more from clinicians and indeed social movements. Networks were at least as important as hierarchies as a mode of mobilizing action. The climate was not 'rationalistic', but rather tinged by waves of panic, guilt and denial.

Ideologically driven change

Alongside the 'new managerialism' of the 1980s arose, perhaps surprisingly, an alternative literature, which advocated a shift of focus from organizational structure to organizational culture. Even more surprisingly, this literature not only gained ground in academic discourse but proved influential with practising managers. Excellent companies, it was claimed (Peters and Waterman 1982), had strong cultures, which could act as organizational glue. The most effective organizational control mechanisms were seen as normative rather than coercive.

Some writers saw symbolic management as a central role of 1980s change agents who were engaged in self-conscious attempts at organizational transformation (Johnson 1990). This signalled a concern with organizational culture in effecting or blocking change. Within established organizational orders, ritual, ceremony and myth may indeed play an important role in giving meaning to a particular paradigm (Pettigrew 1979). Language systems emerge, which frame social life in different ways. In the HIV/AIDS field, new forms of visual imagery also played a key role in sending 'messages' to the audience.

However, two important questions emerge. First, is 'symbolic management' really the conscious preserve of culture changers? This is to take a very plastic and top-down approach to the study of organizational culture. Taking HIV/AIDS as a tracer issue, we can ask whether such symbolic and cultural aspects are indeed being managed deliberately (and if so, by whom) or whether they emerge in a more collective, inchoate and unplanned form.

Second, where do strong organizational cultures come from? It is possible that they are imprinted on an organization, for example, by a strong founder–entrepreneur. But it may be that organizational cultures reflect wider changes to value systems observable in society, or at least certain subcultures. In certain circumstances, the term 'culture', may be too anaemic to capture the true essence of what is in effect a coherent 'ideology', which contains a number of interlinked values and beliefs. There may even be a contest for intellectual hegemony apparent between a number of conflicting ideologies.

The analysis of such an ideologized field of change presents some distinctive challenges, which are rather different from those apparent in the conventional management of change literature. Chapter 3 addresses this question, highlighting the role of social movements in generating new ideologies, which may then become incorporated within formal organizations.

Issue recognition

Many accounts assume that organizational change starts from the need to improve performance within an already identified strategic framework. As a performance gap gradually increases (e.g. progressive loss of financial control), so the need to trigger remedial action grows. This can be seen as a relatively simple organizational change process. Another and more complex type of organizational change – less frequently addressed in the management literature until recently – results from a perception of a need to change in order to address qualitatively different and unexpected events.

Here, as exemplified by the HIV/AIDS issue, the driving force for change comes from outside and intrudes itself on the organization. The organization has little in the way of existing knowledge, templates or decision-making routines to process such potentially threatening issues. In the early 1980s, for example, even the basic epidemiology relating to HIV/AIDS was undeveloped. As a very first step, actors within the organization have to 'sense' the incipient change in the environment and begin to construct this as a legitimate focus for action within the organization.

These questions are addressed in Chapter 5. We are here analysing the initial stages of a long-term change process in which new information is being acquired by organizational actors, which then leads them to embark upon social and organizational action. In analysing this process of becoming aware of HIV/AIDS as an issue, we highlight the role of a small group of clinical academics, other clinicians, and people involved in social movements who, for particular and idiosyncratic reasons, sensed the significance and the urgency of the issue early and took a personal interest.

Entrepreneurial activity, coalition building and crisis management

Entrepreneurial activity and coalition building

Whereas in Chapter 5 we analyse the response of the very early movers in the field in 'sensing' the new HIV/AIDS issue, in Chapter 6 we consider the next stage in the change process: turning awareness into action and building a wider coalition across the organization to support service development. The HIV/AIDS issue involved so many different settings and organizations that forming an interorganizational network was of prime importance.

The problem is that the qualities required of 'product champions' (Rothwell 1976; Stocking 1985), in the problem sensing and coalition building stages of the change process are very different – perhaps even contradictory – in nature. As Downs (1967) points out, bureaucratic organizations contain so much inertia that it may be that only 'zealots' have the obsessive drive and energy to put new issues on agendas; social movement organizations might be thought to be good candidates for undertaking this kind of energy raising activity. So change processes may start with deviants and heretics at the edge of the organization and only slowly work inwards and upwards.

In the later coalition building phase, however, zealotry is less important than diplomacy. Horizontally, there is the need to connect a wide variety of different settings. Vertically, there is a need to connect to power figures and to secure a flow of resources (money, time, attention). This is considered in more detail in Chapter 7 where we consider the role of the 'product champion' in the process of cross-boundary working.

Crisis management

By 1986–87, a full-scale national crisis was being constructed around the HIV/AIDS issue. In this section of the chapter, we are concerned with the role of a perception of crisis in helping a new issue rise up an organization's agenda. As part of this, we address the concept of crisis, how issues come to be seen as crises and the effect of a perception that a crisis exists on the subsequent management of an issue.

It seems that the term 'crisis management' frequently carries pejorative overtones. 'What', it seems to imply, 'was management doing to let this crisis develop? Should it not have intervened before events got out of hand?' The inference is that if only something *had* been done about it earlier, that something would have been more appropriate and more carefully thought out. Is this a fair view to take of the response to the HIV/AIDS epidemic? Or did crisis management in fact provide sources of fluidity, energy and creativity that it would have been difficult to find in non-crisis conditions?

We also look briefly at the opposite process of moving beyond a crisis state. What is the consequence of a 'crisis issue' becoming perceived as of lesser importance, or even being redefined as a non-issue as a result of a view that previous activity had resulted from someone constructing a pseudo-crisis? What happens when there is a move from crisis management to institutionalization, and does this result in a loss of momentum for development and innovation?

There is also a theoretical debate about the nature of managing in a crisis, which we can address using our empirical material. Much of the existing literature on organizational crisis (Hermann 1963; Jick and Murray 1982) stresses the pathological consequences of 'crisis as threat', which may paradoxically reduce the energy, creativity and flexibility so much needed. Within public sector management, Levine et al.'s (1982) analysis of the response within New York City to the fiscal crisis of the mid-1970s found that rapid retrenchment stifled initiative and encouraged errors.

The counter-scenario of 'crisis as opportunity' is less developed, although Starbuck et al. (1978) take up this theme in their paper on three organizations that responded positively to enforced change. Major change is here seen as much more likely to take place when the perception of a crisis forces awkward issues up agendas. The process of strategic change in ICI (Pettigrew, 1985) would be another example where concern about sudden loss of financial performance was the trigger for wider change. Under these conditions very different patterns of organizational behaviour may be present. We are likely to see continuing pressure from pioneers, the formation of special groups that seek to evangelize the rest of the organization, high energy and commitment levels and a period of organizational plasticity in which anything seems possible. There is, therefore, rapid learning, consciousness raising and mobilization. In the health care sector, Meyer's (1982) study of an 'environmental jolt' (an unexpected and unprecedented strike by physicians) suggested that:

> By plunging organizations into unfamiliar circumstances, jolts can legitimate unorthodox experiments that revitalize them, teach lessons that reacquaint them with their environments and inspire dramas celebrating their ideologies.

Working across boundaries

A multiplicity of agencies, settings and professional and occupational groupings quickly became involved in the processing of the HIV/AIDS issue. Nor is it easy to see how this interorganizational complexity could be much reduced, given that HIV/AIDS is a multifaceted syndrome rather than a discrete disease.

The effective crossing of these boundaries represents a key skill in the management of HIV/AIDS services and also an important theme for analysis. A tension is apparent between formal and informal accounts of interorganizational cooperation. Cooperation was mandated from the centre, and formal machinery established. However, there are also important informal organizational processes apparent which shape the extent of joint working achieved, both as facilitators and as inhibitors. In our view, these informal processes were more powerful than the formal processes.

Individual, group and organizational learning

We should consider processes of organizational change in part as a cognitive (Johnson 1990), and indeed as a learning, process. An unfreezing–flux–refreezing model is often used within the management of change literature, with the assumption that, initially, an old paradigm breaks up in response to environmental change. There is then a period of information building, experimentation and flux. Finally a new paradigm will be embedded in the organization as it returns to a new steady state. As Johnson (1990) points out, such models are not informative about the sorts of managerial activities that give rise to these stages or that legitimize information-building or experimentation.

More recently, increasing interest has been shown in the so-called 'learning organization' (Jones and Hendry 1992). This is seen as a new type of organization, which values its staff and seeks to develop them to promote learning, adaptation and change. A number of organizations are now declaring themselves to be 'learning organizations'.

However, such accounts may overconcentrate on the organizational level and falsely assume that the transition from individual to organizational learning is not problematic. In Chapter 8, we question this assumption by examining processes of individual, group and organizational learning around HIV/AIDS. We suggest that there is evidence of widespread learning at individual and small group level. Whether this has translated into 'organizational learning' is quite another question.

Elsewhere we have characterized the NHS as dominated by a culture of short-term panics (Pettigrew et al. 1992). The danger is one of process without memory, and of action without reflection. The obstacles in the way of the construction of a 'learning organization' in the NHS should not be underestimated.

Concluding remarks

The organizational and managerial response to HIV/AIDS is of major societal importance in its own right and as such is worthy of analysis and reflection. We believe furthermore that currently there is an important gap in the HIV/AIDS literature in this area. Key questions revolve around processes of organizational change and resistance to change. How did new service systems emerge? Who provided energy and leadership for change? Who provided counterinterpretations or resisted the direction of development? We see this book as helping to fill this gap in the field.

In addition, HIV/AIDS can act as a 'tracer issue' for a number of broad themes in the literature on organizational change, and we have signalled what these theoretical issues might be in this introductory chapter. We now have a well-developed database of longitudinal and comparative case studies, which can be interrogated in the light of these theoretical themes. After presenting our data, we then return in the final chapter to consider what implications our results might have for the more general literature on organizational change.

HIV/AIDS – a new issue

Introduction

In this chapter, we set the scene for the rest of the book by describing the HIV/AIDS issue and giving an overview of some of the major questions it has raised for groups and organizations concerned. Here, as throughout the book, we focus on developing an organizational analysis of the response to HIV/AIDS in the British context. While there is work on what is seen as the organizational failure of the US health care system to deal appropriately with the issue (e.g. Perrow and Guillen 1990), there is less analysis available of the very different response of the British health care system, where in fact sources of energy were at least as apparent as sources of resistance.

In the previous chapter, we began by conceiving of HIV/AIDS as a health care issue that was processed by a number of very different organizations. It has also been an issue that, arising out of a few obscure cases of immunodeficiency disease, tucked away in a specialist journal, progressed to become *the* public health issue of the 1980s, arousing a massive amount of attention and concern. Government, public and media awareness of the issue was at its peak in the mid-1980s, but since then, for various reasons, the issue has become institutionalized and interest has faded. So, with HIV/AIDS we are looking not just at a specific health care issue, but at the career of a public issue in its organizational context. Indeed, Hogwood (1987) suggests that public issues have distinct careers, often moving from 'crisis to complacency'. Questions of power and the political process also intrude as candidate issues have to fight to get onto public policy agendas, and then to stay there. Issues need friends at court if they are to remain the focus of official attention, and constant issue succession takes place, so that the currently fashionable issue soon becomes unfashionable as the spotlight switches to still newer issues. Issues start by seeming tractable, but become increasingly intractable in their turn. This seems to suggest strong life-cycle effects in the careers of public policy issues.

Nor should we subscribe to the naïve functionalist view that 'necessity is the mother of invention'. Just because HIV/AIDS represented a health care issue and, like most health care issues, a social problem, did not mean that it would necessarily become a public issue. Given the association of HIV/AIDS with traditionally powerless minority groups, perhaps the surprise should be that the issue ever rose so high onto the official policy agenda in the first place, rather than that it failed to stay there.

The first section of this chapter is taken up with a brief description of HIV and AIDS, its transmission characteristics, the history of the discovery of this new health issue and details of the current prevalence of the infection (so far as it is known) in Britain and world-wide.

In the following section we set HIV/AIDS in its historical, social and organizational contexts. Even in a field as apparently 'new' as HIV/AIDS, there are aspects of past history that weigh a heavy hand in terms of both medical culture and a 'folk memory' of responses to previous epidemics. Some prior comparator health care issues are discussed and the concept of 'epidemic psychology' is outlined. We then look briefly at some aspects of British society in the 1970s and early 1980s, such as changing attitudes to sexuality, moves towards promoting individual choice and alternative solutions to institutionalized care and questioning of the primacy of 'scientific' solutions, which all had their effect on the response to HIV. In terms of the organizational context, we look at the ways in which the NHS as a whole was changing in the 1980s and the way in which these changes were one manifestation of the wider political climate of the Thatcher administration.

We then describe, in the third section of the chapter, the 'career' of the HIV/AIDS issue to date, and suggest that this can usefully be divided into three distinct 'periods': prelegitimation; legitimation and postlegitimation.

Medical and epidemiological aspects of the issue

Clinical aspects of the virus

Human immunodeficiency virus (HIV), is a blood borne virus, which progressively destroys the human immune system. The virus is present in the blood and semen of infected people, and may be passed on to others through transference of either of these fluids. The most common modes of transmission of HIV are through sexual intercourse, sharing contaminated injecting equipment, receipt of contaminated blood products and from mother to child during pregnancy.

For a time after infection, possibly for as long as ten years or more, although the presence of HIV can be demonstrated through a blood test, there may be no outward physical indication of this process and, in the absence of other, unrelated, illness the infected person will remain fit and healthy. However, the virus progressively destroys CD4 lymphocytes (a type of white blood cell found in the lymph nodes and spleen), which play a central role in the protective response to the numerous naturally occurring organisms that regularly enter the body, the so-called 'opportunistic' infections. Once the number of CD4 cells decreases below a certain level, symptoms of infection by some of these organisms begin to appear, indicating that the immune system is impaired.

Symptoms are often relatively trivial at first but, over time, the number and severity of episodes of illness increases, leading ultimately to a diagnosis of acquired immune deficiency syndrome (AIDS). Clinically, AIDS manifests itself as a variety of cancers and bacterial, viral and fungal infections. These may affect many different parts of the body, including the skin, lungs, digestive system and central nervous system. There is currently no known cure for AIDS, which, if untreated, leads rapidly to death from overwhelming infection. However, with constantly improving methods of treatment, people with AIDS can live for a number of years.

The HIV pandemic

Although it is now thought possible that human immunodeficiency virus has been around for a long time, possibly even since the 1950s (Corbitt et al. 1990) and certainly since the late 1970s (Adler 1988), the disease now called AIDS was first described as a specific condition affecting gay men in the USA in 1981 (Center for Disease Control 1981).

Initially it was not realized that the condition was caused by a virus, but it rapidly became apparent that similar symptoms were appearing in some people who had been given blood transfusions or blood products. This pointed to an infective agent and, by 1983, the virus had been isolated. The first tests that could detect an antibody response and thus demonstrate the presence of HIV were produced a year later.

Since then many people all over the world have been tested for HIV. None the less, it has been very difficult to get an accurate picture of the prevalence and spread of HIV world-wide. Uptake of voluntary testing programmes has been adversely affected by varying degrees of accessibility in different areas, by the stigma and ostracism experienced by many of those known to be infected and by failure of individuals to identify themselves as having been at risk of acquiring the virus.

To improve epidemiological information there have also been unlinked anonymous testing programmes where blood obtained for other purposes is stripped of any identification before carrying out the test. In some countries there is also mandatory testing of some groups of people, such as those applying for military service.

As well as collecting figures for the number of positive HIV test results, most countries also ask doctors to report cases of AIDS. The World Health Organization collects and collates the reported figures for HIV and AIDS and regularly produces statistics showing the increase and spread of the pandemic (world-wide epidemic). From these figures, they also attempt to estimate the actual prevalence of infection, as the testing and reporting systems are less comprehensive in some countries than in others.

Despite uncertainty about the precise figures involved, however, it is clear that there are different patterns of prevalence in different countries. Sub-Saharan Africa is thought to have the greatest number of cases of infection, and in Africa there are roughly as many females as males with HIV, suggesting that the spread of infection is there predominantly through heterosexual intercourse. This mode of transmission also predominates in other developing countries, such as Asia and Latin America, though they apparently have smaller numbers infected at present. Elsewhere, HIV is currently more prevalent amongst those involved in homosexual intercourse and in sharing injecting equipment.

Current British epidemiology

Figures for the numbers of people in Britain testing positive for HIV infection and of those with diagnoses of AIDS are collected by the Communicable Diseases Surveillance Centre. Although reporting is voluntary, rather than required by law as is the case with many other infectious diseases, in practice it is considered that the degree of under-reporting in Britain is relatively small. Nevertheless, as there are initially no signs of a person having been infected, it is possible that many will not be identified before they develop symptoms, and epidemiologists cannot therefore base predictions of future cases of AIDS directly on projections of known cases of HIV.

Early predictions, notably the Cox Report (DHSS 1988), assumed exponential growth of the number of cases, as had been seen amongst the gay population in North America in the early 1980s, but it is now recognized that conditions for spread of the virus and for the rate of progress to a diagnosis of AIDS have been very different in Britain, not only from that in the USA but also from those obtaining in other European countries and other parts of the world, and some of the reasons for this will be discussed in later chapters. None the less, there has been a continuing, though slower than initially predicted, increase in numbers of cases of HIV infection and AIDS, and the most recent projections for Britain (*The Day Report*; Public Health Laboratory Service 1993) suggest a continuing increase in incidence so that in 1997 there will be around 2400 new reports of cases of AIDS.

An additional complication in making predictions is shifting demographic and geographic variations in incidence of infection. For instance, it was initially assumed that HIV would spread rapidly amongst injecting drug users through needle sharing but, probably mostly as a result of an increase in the availability of clean injecting equipment, the predicted rapid spread has not occurred.

Geographically the first reported cases of HIV infection and AIDS were concentrated in (mainly teaching) hospitals in the major cities, particularly London. This meant that HIV was frequently seen as a minor issue elsewhere. However, this was partly an artifact of the reporting process and of patient mobility, and a combination of structural changes in the National Health Service (NHS) and changing perceptions amongst both patients and doctors about where and how treatment should be delivered is beginning to alter these initial geographic patterns.

The historical, social and organizational contexts in which HIV appeared

A *new epidemic – what histories are repeating themselves?*

HIV/AIDS has marked a return to the 'epidemic' among first-world health care systems that had thought that epidemics that were not readily amenable to medical intervention and limitation were events of the past.

Advances in 'scientific' medicine and the advent of antibiotics and vaccines following the Second World War had spelled the end of wards full of people with syphilis, tuberculosis, poliomyelitis, diphtheria and the various epidemic infectious diseases of childhood. Since then, although there had been a number of new outbreaks of infectious diseases that had briefly captured the headlines, these had either been treated relatively easily, with few fatalities (food poisoning, hepatitis B, meningitis), or posed a threat to fairly restricted numbers of the population (legionnaires' disease, Lassa fever). In fact, not since bubonic plague in the seventeenth century had there been any epidemic that both affected large numbers of people and was almost universally fatal.

The HIV/AIDS epidemic, with no available remedial treatment and preventable only by indirect means rather than directly through vaccination, reactivated spectres from a past still lodged in a collective folk memory based on hearsay and historical accounts of horrific events. In addition, many found the association of the epidemic with long-standing sexual taboos difficult to come to terms with. It is therefore hardly surprising that HIV/AIDS has had a profoundly disorientating effect on both individuals and organizations, leading to knee-jerk reactions characterized by a harking back to the perceived values and attitudes of previous ages in which both 'deviant' sexual behaviours and people suffering from infectious and contagious diseases were regulated by law.

This strong subjective element in the construction of an epidemic and the nature of 'epidemic psychology' (Strong 1990) cries out for analysis. Strong argues that epidemic psychology contains at least three distinct components: (1) fear; (2) explanation/moralization; and (3) calls to action. Epidemics may then mobilize those who have their pet solutions or reform projects to propose, as they suddenly discover new opportunities for action.

Individuals have to devise their stance in relation to the epidemic. Do they deny its existence, treat it as one more issue, or embrace it as of overwhelming importance? Individual 'product champions' – particularly if high status – were of considerable importance in developing services in the localities and some of those we interviewed talked of the moment when they realized that for them HIV/AIDS was going to become of key significance. Other respondents insisted, even in the face of contrary evidence, that the issue was unlikely to affect their particular area of responsibility. Others varied their degree of interest depending on the issue's current visibility in the media and political topicality. We discuss how HIV/AIDS was constructed as an issue in greater detail in Chapter 5.

A changing social and organizational context

Alongside continuity stands change. HIV/AIDS arose at the end of three decades in which there had been rapid social and cultural change. The immediate postwar years of relative privation and hardship had given way to an expanding economy and proliferating educational opportunities, all within the framework of a growing welfare state free at the point of delivery.

In addition, the postwar generation were increasingly questioning of traditional authority and morality, moving towards a culture favouring individual freedom. Increasingly permissive attitudes were particularly noticeable around such previously socially unacceptable behaviours as drug use and sexual liaisons outside marriage. The use of cannabis became almost respectable amongst those espousing the new liberal culture, even those injecting addictive drugs such as heroin came to be viewed as more in need of help and support than prosecution, while the advent of the contraceptive pill encouraged increasing tolerance of multiple and non-traditional sexual relationships, including homosexuality and lesbianism.

Collective social action based on ideological commitment to a particular set or sets of beliefs and values was neither new to this period, nor a purely gay phenomenon. However, as we explore in greater detail in Chapter 3, new social movements and their physical structural manifestations – social movement organizations (SMOs) – were very much part of the culture of this period. Interestingly, the character of the new SMOs, whether espousing the causes of people disadvantaged by disability, race or sexual preference, or promoting 'alternative' lifestyles, therapies or dietary regimes, also reflected the new preoccupations with individual rights and freedoms rather than the collective solidarity of existing movements, such as trades unions.

However, by the beginning of the 1970s it was becoming apparent that the new freedoms and opportunities had brought some problems as well as pleasures, not least amongst them being the spread of infectious diseases hitherto confined to relatively small groups of people. Muraskin (1993) summarizes the position succinctly with reference to the epidemic of hepatitis B which, albeit with less publicity, preceded that of HIV by ten years:

> The hepatitis B epidemic demonstrated the existence of a series of infectious super 'highways'; transmission routes paved by major social, technological and cultural changes: increased medical innovations requiring significant exposure to blood, sexual revolution (straight and gay), large scale recreational and addictive drug use and massive international travel. Looking at that new thoroughfare one could predict that other diseases would ultimately come rolling down it.

As well as fostering the formation of new SMOs, the permissive climate of the 1960s and 1970s also affected the policies followed by many existing organizations, from the government downwards. In particular the Labour Party, in power for most of this period, with its tradition of being the platform for the oppressed and underprivileged, had been responsible for most of the liberalizing legislation, for increased public sector spending and for policies of support for minority groups.

However, by the end of the 1970s the climate of public opinion was changing. Increasing financial problems had already forced restrictions on spending in general, and health service spending in particular, and a new Conservative government, with a rhetorical commitment to reinstating 'Victorian values' had, according to Strong and Robinson (1990): 'Rejected, in principle at least, not merely the work of one, two or three decades but of almost the whole century.'

Amongst the changes instituted by the Thatcher regime was a re-emphasis on law and order, including the role of the police in apprehending and prosecuting people using illegal drugs (this was later seen by some as having increased needle sharing in some areas, leading to the spread of HIV). In addition, a rejection of the permissive sexual culture led to a reexamination of public sector support for the gay movement and of sex education in schools. Here there was a re-emphasis on the conventional family unit and more power for school governors in deciding what children should learn about sex and when. This supported those who felt that sex education had become too explicit and had placed insufficient emphasis on moral standards and has led in some schools to a degree of deliberalization of sex education. As Clift and Stears (1991), commenting on research into HIV/AIDS education in schools, point out, such attitudes may complicate efforts to teach effectively about contraception and sexually transmitted diseases, including HIV/AIDS.

The government also began to institute far-reaching changes in the NHS, aimed at stemming the increasing amount of public money being spent on it by infusing into it private sector concepts of management such as management by objectives, efficiency, value for money and competitive tendering for service contracts. Area Health Authorities (AHAs) were abolished, reducing the tiers of management from three to two, and general management was introduced, with an influx of new personnel from the private sector. This process continued throughout the 1980s with a further reorganization in 1989, instituting an internal market for services through a split between the purchaser and provider functions.

Although all these changes had no direct effect on HIV/AIDS, which became a major health issue during this period, there were a number of indirect effects, not least in diverting the attention of managers from the issue.

The career of the HIV/AIDS issue

The history of the organizational response to HIV/AIDS as a new health issue for Britain can be usefully analysed as having three 'stages': (1) a prelegitimation stage (roughly, 1981–86); (2) a legitimation stage (1986–87); and (3) a postlegitimation stage (1987 onwards). The cast of decision makers involved can be seen as changing from one 'stage' to another. We will develop this argument further in later chapters, but here it is sufficient to describe its general structure.

The prelegitimation period

At first, following recognition of the new disease, action within the official health care system was limited to a few specialist academic doctors and clinicians who were early in anticipating that the increasing numbers of patients seen in the USA would soon be paralleled in Britain, and used their relative autonomy to acquire funding to set up research studies.

There were also early approaches to management about the need for more beds for immunocompromised patients (Ferlie and Pettigrew 1988). Nevertheless, it is probably true to say that most NHS managers (who in any case were preoccupied with major reorganizations and the introduction of general management) saw AIDS as no more than a newly identified disease affecting a particular group of patients, but with only marginal consequences for their organizations.

Outside the NHS, however, members of the gay community in Britain were shocked by some of the early deaths from AIDS. They recognized, far sooner than the government and most of the medical establishment, that this was going to be a major health problem here as well as in the USA, and in 1983 they started the first voluntary organization dedicated to educating about AIDS and supporting those infected, the Terrence Higgins Trust (THT), based in central London.

Initially at least, THT's organizational culture was clearly that of an SMO – radical and campaigning with a commitment to furthering gay rights, protecting confidentiality of people with HIV and lobbying the government to take the issue on board. It achieved a surprising degree of respectability for such an organization, mostly because it quickly became recognized as the only authoritative voice on many of the personal and social issues raised by the epidemic. In addition, as Schramm-Evans (1990) points out, during the early 1980s, before the government had committed itself publicly to addressing the issue, by granting the organization relatively small sums of money it was able to use THT to promote policies with which it would otherwise have had difficulty in being associated.

Although THT was formally the first, other similar (if smaller) gay voluntary organizations were quickly formed in other areas and made efforts to influence local authorities and health services to take the issue seriously and develop what they felt were appropriate policies on prevention and care issues. Their degree of success, and the influence they exerted, particularly on local authorities, during those early years, tended to be very dependent on the local political climate.

Within the NHS, at least some of those who were dealing with HIV-infected patients were aware of social pressures from these outside organizations and receptive to their concerns. However, it was the discovery in 1983 that AIDS was caused by an infectious virus that marked the beginning of a specifically managerial response to HIV/AIDS as an issue for the whole of the NHS, rather than relating solely to a few patients on a ward.

First, there was an explosion of media interest, followed by considerable concern about the possible transmission of infection from patients to hospital staff. There were instances of some staff in hospitals where there were known to be cases of AIDS threatening industrial action and taking extreme protective precautions. Working parties were urgently convened to produce comprehensive guidelines for staff dealing with infected patients, and hospitals also started to look critically and urgently at their control of infection procedures. The sense of caution and commitment to avoiding cross-infection, which had been instilled into nursing and medical staff trained before the days of vaccines and antibiotics, had gradually attenuated over twenty years of simple and effective treatments for infections. Many hospitals found that standards for even ordinary cleanliness had fallen and that major investment was required to achieve appropriate standards of hygiene and sterility for wards and operating theatres.

It was also at this stage that the government began to get involved with the issue, with concerns about possible contamination of blood supplies prompting publication of a government leaflet in September 1983 (DHSS 1983a) exhorting prospective donors who thought they could be at risk from AIDS not to donate blood. In addition, health authorities were issued with the first control of infection guidelines on AIDS from the Advisory Committee on Dangerous Pathogens.

The early impact of the discovery of AIDS and HIV on the main medical specialties (genitourinary medicine, drugs services, haemophilia and infectious diseases) now most closely involved in the identification and treatment of HIV infection, varied. Some of the reasons for this are embedded in the historical development of the specialties and are discussed at greater length in Chapter 3, but individual clinicians in the different specialties were also divided in their perception of the importance of this new issue. Patients showing symptoms of AIDS and AIDS-related illness usually required inpatient treatment and went to infectious diseases units. However, the early cases were mostly confined to London, though other areas with a substantial gay community, such as Manchester, also had patients. Clinicians dealing with people with AIDS soon recognized the importance of this new disease, but genitourinary medicine departments, where most people with HIV are now seen on an outpatient basis long before they require admission, do not usually have inpatient beds, and inpatient units for infectious diseases tended to be provided on a regional basis, so most hospitals had no patients at all for a long time. A few clinicians in genitourinary medicine were notable for their interest in and commitment to the issue even in the absence of patients, but these were few and far between.

Where drugs services were concerned, despite the fact that AIDS was already being diagnosed amongst drug users in the USA, at this early stage few of those dealing with problems of addiction saw AIDS as a problem that might concern their patients. This was partly because the first reports of AIDS affecting drug users did not get nearly so much publicity as the epidemic amongst gay men, and also because drugs services in Britain were, in the main, focused on those patients who were prepared to cooperate with a programme of abstinence. Those who wished to continue to inject were therefore not defined as patients.

Public health doctors were another group who might have been expected to take an interest in AIDS. Some certainly took a keen interest from very early on, and the chief medical officer in the Department of Health, Sir Donald Acheson, has been praised for taking the issue seriously far sooner than some of those in similar positions in other countries (Berridge and Strong 1992). However, public health is a very broad field and many public health physicians were (and continue to be) more concerned about such issues as heart disease and smoking, which currently cause far more ill-health in the general population than HIV.

On the other hand, physicians in the regional haemophilia centres became concerned about HIV from very early on. Britain, though more or less self-sufficient for supplies of whole blood, did not produce sufficient Factor VIII, the clotting factor needed by people with haemophilia. A dose of Factor VIII is derived from many separate donations of blood, and much of the shortfall was imported from the USA, where reports were now suggesting that much of their donated blood had been contaminated. Details of the first case of AIDS in a haemophiliac in Britain were published in October 1983, but even before then, the directors of the ten haemophilia 'reference centres', which offer specialist advice and help to the other 110 haemophilia centres throughout the country, had drafted guidelines on the use of blood products and how to counsel patients.

With the virus identified and anxieties about the safety of blood supplies increasing, producing a diagnostic test for the virus, which could be used on a large scale, was a high priority. By mid-1984, various prototype tests were available and, by 1985, the government was advocating the setting up of separate testing sites to avoid the blood transfusion services from becoming overwhelmed by requests for tests from those who thought they might have been infected.

The advent of testing finally delivered incontrovertible proof of the spread of HIV infection. As anticipated by those already working in the field, many people who had up to then shown no symptoms suggestive of AIDS were found to be carrying HIV. These included many of the people in Britain with haemophilia, and many more gay men. The major surprise, however, came from Scotland where a virologist in Edinburgh, trying out the test on stored samples of sera taken from injecting drug users, discovered that an unexpectedly large number of these were also infected with HIV. This was the finding that, above all others, finally convinced the government that action must be taken. Until that point, it had been possible for some to argue that, now that blood donors were tested, and supplies of Factor VIII were being heat-treated, the epidemic had been contained and the infection was only likely to spread amongst gay men, seen as a marginal group. With the realization that many drug users were infected there was immediate concern that they could act as a vector for spreading HIV into the heterosexual community.

Legitimating HIV/AIDS

With the recognition of the possibility of heterosexual spread, it was no longer possible to ignore the threat posed by the epidemic and, from then onwards, the HIV/AIDS issue became officially recognized and legitimated by the British Government. The issue of government booklets on AIDS to the general public in 1984, was quickly followed up by the formation of a House of Commons Select Committee enquiry into AIDS, provision of special money for those London hospitals with the greatest numbers of patients, the setting up of dedicated testing clinics and a massive country-wide health education campaign.

There was also a structural response to the issue. An AIDS unit was set up in the prestigious Department of Health offices in Whitehall, an AIDS unit formed an important part of the newly instituted Health Education Authority and, in 1986, an official directive went to district and regional health authorities to appoint named physicians (in most cases from public health) for HIV/AIDS and to set up local committee structures chaired by them for dealing with the issue.

This decision to impose formal structures from the top was one that had important consequences on the subsequent development of services. The directive was, in essence, a public health physician's charter, signalling that they were expected to take over the managerial reins, if that were not already the case, and reflecting the increasing status of these doctors inside a progressively more managerially orientated health service. Such a change of lead had three main effects: (1) it re-emphasized HIV/AIDS as a medical issue; (2) it gave a new impetus to prevention; and (3) it created a bureaucratic buffer between clinicians championing the cause and general management, at district and regional level.

Once structural support for the issue was assured, government money started to flow ever more freely, although it was not until 1988 that the principle of ring-fenced funding for a wide spectrum of HIV/AIDS services, distributed to districts by regions, became established. Prior to that, the money made available for particular developments was essentially based on the efforts of lobbyists with particular interests. Hence, as well as support for the London hospitals with large numbers of patients, there was a mushrooming of 'counselling' appointments, based on a developing ideology, particularly within the voluntary sector, of the 'correct' way to deal with people wanting to be tested and those found to be HIV positive and needing further support and help.

In addition, drugs services, already receiving pump-priming money as part of the government's campaign against drug use, now argued that the only way to prevent even more drug users becoming infected was to provide clean injecting equipment. This was a controversial view, but the evidence from Scotland, laid out in the McClelland Report (SHHD 1986), convinced the government to institute pilot needle exchange schemes.

It should be noted that all this legitimating activity was instituted on the basis of belief in the reality of the problem, rather than accurate knowledge. Actual evidence of the prevalence and incidence of HIV infection was even more scanty then than it is now, and the first set of epidemiological projections, which assumed large exponential increases in numbers of people with AIDS over the next few years (*the Cox Report*; DHSS 1988), were based on a very small number of actual cases collected over a very short period. Nevertheless, although the authors of the report clearly stated the uncertain nature of their predictions, the period between 1985 and 1987 was one in which HIV/AIDS was hyped into a crisis, essentially as a result of a combination of media attention, lobbying by special interest groups and the intervention of government officials and committees, including one at Cabinet level (this last despite what Street (1993) argues was a lack of interest in the issue by the head of government, Margaret Thatcher).

Postlegitimation period

HIV/AIDS was now 'official', and organizational structures were developing. In addition, one-off resources for HIV were increasing rapidly and there were plans to formalize funding by 'ring-fencing' a special government allocation, a policy that went right against general health service funding policy and indicated the degree to which government had been convinced of overwhelming need.

As well as funding a diversity of specific schemes, often aimed at prevention, increasing funding meant the possibility of actually employing people to deal specifically with particular aspects of the issue. Money for counselling led to counselling posts, money for prevention to the employment of health educators and the perceived necessity for coordination of services led to some authorities taking the lead in employing people with this specific remit. These HIV coordinators were frequently recruited from the voluntary sector, now made respectable by official government policy.

In a health service that had felt itself to be increasingly starved of money over the previous decade the 'new' money did not go unnoticed and there was no shortage of proposals on how to spend it. These ranged from proposals to open million pound plus 'AIDS units' and outpatients clinics put forward by specialties such as infectious diseases and genitourinary medicine (who were usually at the bottom of the list when it came to improvements); through requests for funds to support a diversity of posts, such as infection control staff, which could be argued to have a link, however small, with HIV; to multitudinous requests for technical items, such as endoscopy equipment, with only the most tenuous connection with HIV/AIDS.

The size of the first ring-fenced allocation, which arrived in 1988–89, was somewhat disappointing, as it was based on numbers of patients with AIDS, and so represented very small amounts of money in most health authorities. However in 1989, central funding for HIV/AIDS was unexpectedly doubled, with some authorities receiving more than five times the previous year's figure, and even district action committees with well-developed plans for future expansion found difficulty in spending all the money immediately.

Paradoxically, the arrival of the big money, for which those convinced of the crucial importance of HIV/AIDS had been lobbying for so long, coincided with the first indications that public and government interest in the HIV/AIDS issue had begun to decline.

The exceptionally high levels of activity around HIV/AIDS, which characterized the mid-1980s were always going to be difficult to sustain indefinitely and it was perhaps inevitable that, following the period of legitimation, a period of normalization and routinization should ensue. Nevertheless, some particular and unforeseen circumstances hastened this process.

The first was the advent, in 1989, of the White Paper *Working for Patients* (Cm 555 1989), which heralded arguably the most radical NHS reorganization since its inception, splitting health authorities into purchasing and providing functions and creating an internal market for services. Not only did this divert general management attention, pushing HIV/AIDS, rarely of major interest, even further down their agendas, but many managers were also faced with considerable financial problems because of the government's insistence on health authorities balancing their books in the run up to implementation.

Even more tellingly, by 1989 it was becoming apparent that numbers of cases of HIV infection and AIDS were not rising as rapidly as the Cox Report had predicted. With the publication of a more restrained set of predictions in the *Day Report* (Public Health Laboratory Service 1990), the voices suggesting that there had been an element of 'crying wolf' seemed suddenly to be drowning those advocating further expansion. There was increasing talk of 'normalizing' the previously abnormal HIV/AIDS issue. A number of hard-pressed NHS general managers also took advantage of the change in public opinion to attempt to vire some of the HIV/AIDS allocation to address what they saw as more important matters:

> The health authority has terrific financial problems, and in a scale of priorities if we didn't have that money earmarked for AIDS we probably wouldn't want to use it in that way . . . There are all kinds of tensions in making money available for something so specifically . . . we all tend to think that AIDS isn't really much of a problem yet, so we will wait until it is and then we will do something about it.

Indeed, the HIV/AIDS budget was a major source of growth in the 1980s in generally hard-pressed budgets in inner city areas, and was sometimes seen as raidable. The 'borrowed' ring-fenced money was soon reclaimed, but the National Audit Office (1991) investigation that brought this issue to public attention also highlighted less overt, but still considerable, misapplication of what some were now seeing as somewhat over-generous funds.

In addition to all this, the voluntary sector, which had advocated so strongly for HIV in the early days, had itself become institutionalized, with large amounts of government funding necessitating the creation of more formal and bureaucratic administrative systems, which alienated some of their members (Schramm-Evans 1990). Torn by internal strife, their influence on government was diminished, further reducing the profile of the issue.

By the early 1990s, though officially HIV/AIDS was still a high priority with government, there were a number of subtle indicators that the issue had, in fact, lost some of its momentum. The AIDS unit was moved from Whitehall to more spacious but less prestigious accommodation south of the river and further away from ministers, the Health Education Authority AIDS unit was wound up, on the grounds that HIV should be seen as part of an overall approach to sexual health and, at district level, although HIV coordinators had been appointed almost everywhere, many found it difficult to achieve the degree of status and influence enjoyed by some of their earlier predecessors.

On the other hand, despite some loss of public interest, the activity of the previous decade had brought some considerable advances. Most major organizations in the public sector now had official HIV/AIDS policies. Prevention activity was continuing, though less high profile and targeted more at those perceived to be at risk. Research was indicating that fewer than expected people who injected drugs were acquiring HIV, almost certainly reflecting the success of the policy to make clean equipment readily available. The importance of having facilities widely available to treat and educate to prevent sexually transmitted diseases of all kinds had been recognized in the *Monks Report* (Department of Health 1988) and considerable resources had been made available to increase and upgrade genitourinary medicine departments. Finally, although no cure for HIV was yet on the horizon, treatments were now available that would enable those with symptoms of HIV to live longer and have a better quality of life than had previously been possible.

Conclusions

In this chapter, we have outlined the natural history of the HIV/AIDS issue in Britain. From obscure beginnings, it briefly came to dominate the politics of health care in 1986–87 before fading as new issues came along in their turn. One might have thought that, given the association of the issue with traditionally marginal and powerless social groupings, and the right-wing political economy of the 1980s, the HIV/AIDS problem would have been ignored by the official policy-making system. However, unlike the situation in the USA, where many have seen the administration as having taken little interest in the issue (Shilts 1987; Perrow and Guillen 1990), in Britain the politics of attention were at least as evident as the politics of neglect.

So far our perspective has been confined to the national policy-making level. Yet services are of course delivered in particular settings in the localities. In the next chapter, therefore, we adopt a more micro perspective, describing and analysing the key service settings that were mobilized in response to the epidemic. From an organization theoretic perspective, it is important to note that these settings are embedded in a variety of different organizational forms (e.g. professionalized bureaucracy, voluntary organizations, social movement organizations). It is also of interest to explore the balance between continuity and change within each setting. In some ways, the impact of the HIV/AIDS issue can be seen as decisive in reshaping – and upgrading – particular settings. In other ways, it reawoke half-submerged folk memories. The HIV/AIDS issue was not always as 'new' as it might superficially appear.

HIV/AIDS and some key service settings

Introduction

In Chapter 2, we suggested that the national 'career' of the HIV/AIDS issue could be seen as having had three stages: (1) prelegitimation; (2) legitimation; and (3) postlegitimation. In this chapter we will take a more microlook at the characteristics of key service settings.

In so doing we need to consider not only the three 'stages' already identified, but a fourth, earlier period, reaching back in some instances long before the beginning of this century, during which services developed the individual characteristics that were later to have a critical impact on their response to HIV/AIDS. The need to include this historical perspective in the analysis of organizational change processes is a fundamental tenet of contextualism, the theoretical orientation underpinning all the research on which this book is based. The rationale for taking this approach has been recently restated by Pettigrew (1990), who warns of the dangers of viewing causation of change as either linear or singular and speaks of the necessity for recognizing the role of history and social processes and the need to identify continuity as well as change in any explanation of contemporary events.

Sarason (1976) also emphasized the importance of historical antecedents in his exploration of the creation of service settings in health care. Using a 'lifecycle' frame of analysis he looked at the experience of small professional groups trying to create and deliver new models of care, especially in the fields of mental health and learning disability. He noted that new settings always arose in some relation to existing settings and that these exerted a crucial influence on the new organization's future development. He also noted that initial optimism often gave way to pessimism, and innovation to routinization, and he was sceptical of the potential for long-term success. This outcome he saw largely as a result of the persistence of sociopolitical relationships, which adversely affected the continuation of the original sense of purpose and mission. His analysis directs our attention to the micropolitics of the organization and how they develop through time.

We can also examine the nature of decision-making processes in the new field of HIV/AIDS. Alford (1975), for instance, suggested that the politics of health care are generally characterized by three blocs: (1) a dominant medical bloc; (2) a challenging managerial bloc; and (3) a repressed community bloc. We can ask whether this analysis fits the new HIV/AIDS field, or whether there are changes in the expected configuration of forces:

1 We will distinguish between settings embedded within professionalized organizations and those springing from different consensus or conflict traditions within the voluntary sector.
2 We describe the historical development of the particular existing settings within health, social services and the voluntary sector that were to be affected by HIV/AIDS.
3 We look at the newly created organizational settings, many of them emerging from a radical social movement tradition, which were triggered by a recognition of the issue.

Different types of settings

The settings from which the new services for HIV/AIDS emerged sprang from two fundamentally different types of organization: (1) statutory sector organizations, such as health and social services, established, legitimated and professionalized with any original radical underpinnings[1] lost in the mists of time; and (2) voluntary sector organizations, often emerging directly from various social movements.

Statutory sector organizations

Professionalized settings
Many service settings that were significant in generating a response to HIV/AIDS were not new or created from lay grass roots, but were already established and professionalized. Such settings display a long history, a given set of power relations and established patterns of belief, and might therefore be seen as less receptive contexts for change (Pettigrew et al.

1992) than more recently established social movement and voluntary organizations. Established settings were certainly subjected to powerful influences for change as a result of the advent of HIV/AIDS (received models of care in drugs services, for instance, were profoundly affected by the epidemic and staff were asked to perform ideological somersaults), but there were also important legacies from the past.

Second, health and social services are professionalized settings. Medicine is often seen as an ideal typical profession, which has legitimated its claims to expertise and autonomy, and this is even more the case for doctors in teaching hospitals at the top of the medical status hierarchy. For Mintzberg (1989), the hospital can be seen as the archetype of the professionalized organization, which is often in a state of perpetual change at a micro level (as knowledgeable medical professionals develop practice) but which is also extremely stable at a strategic level.

Unlike medicine, the claims to professional status of other groups in the health service, such as nurses, physiotherapists, health promotion officers, and social workers, has been a subject for debate. Toren (1969) for instance described social work and nursing as, by strict functionalist definition, only semiprofessions. Becker (1962), however, suggested that 'professional' is more usefully thought of as symbolic of a particular sort of activity, while Freidson (1970) defines a profession as an occupation dominating a division of labour with its claim to special status recognized by the state. Nurses, physiotherapists and social workers certainly fulfil these criteria, and all these groups are increasingly seen as having a considerable degree of autonomy in certain situations. The Aves report (Aves 1969), which considers the relationship between volunteers and professional social workers, lists the functions of social workers as including development and implementation of policy, diagnosis of problems and management. These groups thus fulfil many criteria of professionalism, and while there may be some debate concerning their status in a continuously developing process of professionalization (Heraud 1978), it is clear from our data that both hospital and social work staff were viewed as part of the professional, statutory response to HIV/AIDS, and distinctively different from the non-statutory sector.

Social movements in professionalized settings
The previous section suggested that there may be a problem about how to secure strategic change across the organization within stable professionalized settings. However, the advent of HIV/AIDS has initiated major changes, aspects of which have affected these organizations right across the board. We need to ask, therefore, what mechanisms were involved, and we suggest that the answer may at least partly lie in Bucher and Strauss' (1961) conceptualization of specialties and 'segments' (specialities in development) within medicine as analogous to social movements.

In contrast to a functionalist sociology of professions, which stressed their cohesiveness and developed form of social organization, they saw professions as loose amalgamations of segments with separate organizational identities, missions and ideologies, pursuing their different objectives in different manners and only held together with some effort.

Not all specialties have equivalent status and differences in standing are one source of the intersegment conflict stressed by Bucher and Strauss (1961) and elaborated in Bucher and Stelling (1977). However, a weakness in Bucher and Strauss' account is that they do not really consider questions of cooperation and coalition forming across segment boundaries, except to reject a simplistic notion of the universality of professional 'colleagueship'. Bucher and Stelling (1977) do identify some mechanisms for integration, as there is continuous face-to-face bargaining between the factions, a search for allies and for compromise and a norm of gentlemanly (*sic*) behaviour; but it may also be important in considering the process of development of services for HIV/AIDS to recognize some more pragmatic reasons for cooperation. Kinston (1983) makes this very clear, pointing out that there is a necessity to share technological resources, diagnostic services, ancillary staff and, of course, patients who are referred between specialist staff as and when required.

There are thus two models of intersegment or interspecialty relationships, one emphasizing the rivalries and power struggles that exist and another concentrating on various mechanisms that favour cooperation. However, as Mintzberg (1989) argues, it may be unnecessary and misleading to see the two models, political or collegial, as existing in isolation:

> Neither common interest nor self interest will dominate decision processes all the time; some combination is naturally to be expected. Professionals may agree on goals yet conflict over how they should be achieved; alternatively consensus can sometimes be achieved even where goals differ . . . Political success sometimes requires a collegial posture – one must cloak self interest in the mantle of the common good. Likewise, collegial ends sometimes require political means.

Much of the previous discussion about professional segments in medicine is also applicable to other professional groups within hospitals, and also to social work. For instance, nurses are also increasingly separated into specialties (e.g. intensive care, paediatrics), while in social work, despite moves to try to reverse the process of specialization, there are strong countervailing influences towards differentiation into specialties (e.g. childcare, mental health). Like medicine, these specialties have explicit and implicit status hierarchies, though in social work these are more linked to the content of the work they undertake than the different client groups they deal with. For instance residential and community workers have much lower status than field (case) workers.

However, although they have a degree of autonomy over how they carry out their individual roles, it is doubtful if other hospital workers and social workers in the different specialisms and segments have as much freedom to devise new ways of working in response to need as doctors do, and this limits the possibility of drawing the same analogy with social movements. There is a more specific division of labour within social work and nursing, with higher status workers taking a purely managerial role and only more junior staff actually dealing directly with clients. This contrasts with the medical hierarchy, where the highest status and most powerful people – the consultants – though they may increasingly have a managerial function, also work closely with patients.

Voluntary sector organizations

Settings based in social movement organizations

Although it may be possible to see some characteristics of specialties within medicine as analogous to SMOs, the best examples of such organizational forms in relation to HIV/AIDS are found in the voluntary sector. As noted in the introduction, Alford (1975) saw the community influence on health care generally as repressed. However, the voluntary sector has gained more status and power over recent years through a combination of increasing acceptance by government of the role of voluntary organizations in providing services that it was unable or unwilling to fund through the state welfare system (Gladstone 1979), and an upsurge in more campaigning forms of community action via 'pressure' groups.

It is this latter form of voluntary action, delivered through the medium of SMOs emerging from the gay liberation movement, which was at first most influential in the development of services for HIV/AIDS; though, as we shall see later, the model of voluntary/statutory collaboration, supported by government, which was the vision of the Wolfenden Committee (1977), has to a great extent diluted and replaced that early radicalism.

SMOs are very different in form and function from classic Weberian bureaucracies (e.g. governmental bureaux). They are above all value-laden organizations concerned about lifestyles, often translating what has hitherto been seen as the personal into the political through tactics of consciousness-raising and group mobilization. A shared ideology may bind a social movement together and a strong group consciousness may develop (see Chapter 4 for a discussion of the wider effects of ideologies in developing services for HIV/AIDS).

SMOs may produce a distinct organizational form and ideological base: a large cultural component, an emphasis on the creation of 'free space', a preference for networks over hierarchies, the possible use of direct action and the linkage of personal experience to drives for collective social change. They in effect act as a vehicle for group mobilization.

The SMOs in this account are also – in Sarason's terms – 'new' settings in that they were organizations newly founded to respond to the HIV/AIDS epidemic, and not (at least initially) highly professionalized. Certainly in their early charismatic period, they reflected the energy and commitment of lay volunteers, themselves often drawn from the communities most affected by the epidemic. However, there may be strong lifecycle effects apparent within SMOs so that the level of energy is raised, but cannot be sustained, leading to burn-out and withdrawal. Associated with this may be a tendency to routinization and the emergence of bureaucratic roles and offices, whereby many of the fluid characteristics listed above fade with the passage of time.

This effect may have been amplified in the case of HIV/AIDS, by the nature of the organizations changing. This happened for a number of reasons to do with sources of funding and the need to present a more 'acceptable' image, as well as the merging of a number of different ideologies, some of which came from a consensus rather than a conflict tradition (McCarthy and Wolfson 1992; see discussion in Chapter 4). However, the consequence was a far-reaching organizational transition from the early community-based groups operating in the field of HIV/AIDS (1981–85) to the quite new configuration of the 'AIDS Service Organizations' (1985 onwards). Patton's (1990) critical account of this transition draws clear links between changes in organizational form and the vagueness or precision of role definitions:

> The new industry developed a vision of itself and of AIDS work that stood in sharp contrast to the early community activism, in which there were few distinctions between organizers, activists, people living with AIDS, and sympathetic medical workers. It inscribed a rigid role structure which constructed 'victims', 'experts' and 'volunteers' as the dramatis personae in the story of AIDS.

Non-SMO voluntary sector settings
Not all voluntary sector settings involved with AIDS sprang from the gay movement, however. Some were 'consumer' groups (e.g. the haemophilia society), others had their roots in the charitable tradition of organizations such as the Church, others still could be seen as the voluntary arms of statutory organizations (e.g. voluntary drugs services).

These could not, strictly, be characterized as SMOs. Morris (1992) argues that the only fruitful way of conceptualizing social movements is in terms of a struggle against systems and structures of domination, and although over time some acquired a more radical and campaigning stance than they had to begin with, their roots were in a consensus, rather than a conflict tradition of voluntary action (McCarthy and Wolfson 1992). Voluntary organizations, after all, have long been seen as, quite simply, a vehicle by which society is enabled to make a more rapid and flexible response to urgent need than is possible for bureaucratic state agencies (Wolfenden Committee 1977, Wilson 1992), and though their ability to carry out this function has been questioned (Kingsley 1981), their role in representing wide agreement over what *should* be done has not.

Sometimes, with established voluntary organizations, lines of demarcation between them and statutory organizations dealing with the same client groups were blurred. Contrary to the usual assumption that voluntary organizations arise organically from within the general population and pioneer new services, it is by no means uncommon, and could be demonstrated even within our relatively small sample, to find that professionals already running statutory sector services also initiate voluntary organizations in order to provide extra help for their client group. This makes for some complex relationships, as suggested by the following comment from a drugs services consultant:

> the [health service drug dependency clinic] is still within the campus of the hospital . . . [the voluntary residential unit] was outside of the health service and we had to have a voluntary management committee and we had to be involved in finding people to run it . . . This all sounds very inbred somehow or other, but it is very important to have management committees in sympathy with what you are doing and a lot were my old Rotary friends who had already been involved in the hospital.

It was some time, as we saw in the last chapter, until HIV/AIDS became seen as a legitimate field of activity, and although some of the earlier voluntary organizations of this type certainly helped to form as well as respond to public opinion, organizations emerging from a consensus tradition were slower to make an impact than their more radical voluntary sector counterparts, possibly because of their links with statutory services and their dependence on them for grant aid. However, as we shall see in the following sections, they have made a distinctive contribution to the development of services for HIV/AIDS and their influence is arguably increasing rather than diminishing as the issue becomes institutionalized.

The effect of different settings on HIV/AIDS service development

In this section we start by considering the historical development of the key statutory sector organizations prior to HIV/AIDS, and how these historic influences affected their response to the issue, before turning to the voluntary sector response, with less of an organizational history behind it, but also playing a crucial role in the development of services.

PreHIV/AIDS – Key professionalized settings

Medical specialties

As far as medical specialties are concerned, HIV/AIDS, initially at least, had hardly any impact on some, while its effect on others has been so great as to change them out of all recognition. Those most closely involved with the HIV/AIDS issue to date have been, on the clinical side, genitourinary medicine, infectious diseases and the haemophilia and drugs services; and one non-clinical specialty – public health. Sometimes there were already established linkages between groupings, for others this was not the case, and individual specialties had developed from quite different traditions. However, there was one linking factor that, though clearly coincidental, was of considerable importance in terms of the response to HIV/AIDS; they could all be seen as, to some extent, 'Cinderella specialties' within the health service hierarchy, relatively marginal and powerless as against the traditional concerns of acute sector medicine and surgery, often not (at least prior to HIV/AIDS) representing attractive career options for medical professionals.

The historical development of these key service settings is crucial to an understanding of the response to HIV/AIDS. The specialty of infectious diseases has perhaps the longest history, with its roots in the old isolation hospitals of the eighteenth and nineteenth centuries, when few effective treatments for even common infections were available and management was focused on prevention of spread of infection. In consequence, from very early on there was a close association between infectious diseases (including sexually transmitted diseases) and public health. This association was institutionalized following the Public Health Act in 1875, when Medical Officers of Health based in local authority departments were given overall responsibility for the running of most hospital and clinic services. The Medical Officer of Health role thus had a long history within local government, and brought together a traditional concern with communicable disease with an interest in the making of 'policy' at a broad level.

However, at the inception of the NHS in 1948, clinical specialties became the responsibility of hospital boards, separating the management of infectious diseases from the public health function, and marking, according to the Acheson Report (DHSS 1988), the beginning of 'a process of debilitation of the specialty of public health medicine'. This hiving-off of responsibilities was followed in the 1974 NHS and local authority reorganization by the splitting of public health into local authority-based environmental health departments, headed by a single Medical Officer of Environmental Health with other public health doctors relocated within the NHS to form departments of community medicine. The new breed of community physicians became members of the post-1974 multidisciplinary consensus teams, though their impact was patchy and somewhat disappointing:

> In some parts of the country, community physicians seized the opportunity which was presented to them in 1974 and created vigorous departments which continue to make important contributions to the planning and development of health services for the populations they serve. In other places they simply failed to make the transition.
>
> (Cm 289 1988: para 2.6)

However, structural problems were not the only reason for the decline of public health. Their major professional expertise had traditionally been in the area of epidemiology and control of infection, and infectious diseases were themselves in decline following the advent of antibiotics and vaccines. The old, isolated fever hospitals, where previously whole wards had been set aside for the treatment of one specific illness, such as syphilis, diphtheria or poliomyelitis, had become monuments to a bygone era. By the 1960s, many hospitals had only one ward set aside for dealing with infectious cases, and the aura of fear and apprehension that had surrounded the specialty was rapidly becoming no more than a folk memory. Treatment and cure was so simple and swift in most instances that a somewhat cavalier attitude had developed generally towards preventing spread of infection.

This attitude was typified by the stance that had begun to be taken by many, particularly in the gay community, to sexually transmitted diseases – that they were simply a readily curable health hazard of a permissive approach to casual sex:

> The fight against venereal disease was proving a Sisyphean task . . . It was now proven statistically that a gay man had one chance in five of being infected with the Hepatitis B virus within twelve months of stepping off the bus into a typical urban gay scene. Within five years infection was a virtual certainty . . . At the New York Gay Men's Health Project, where Dan William was medical director, 30 percent of the patients suffered from gastro-intestinal parasites . . . he had his 'regulars' who came in with infection after infection, waiting for the magic bullet.
>
> (Shilts 1987: 18–19)

This upfront and casual approach to sexually transmitted diseases was very different from the one long associated with genitourinary medicine, whose patients had been a stigmatized group and whose 'clap' doctors themselves had been stigmatized by association. Historically, such diseases had been associated with a complex mixture of moral, social, public health and indeed political issues and had involved a tendency to apportion 'blame' in the transmission of infection, leading to recurrent attempts to regulate forms of sexual deviance such as promiscuity, prostitution and homosexuality.

The old voluntary hospitals were often reluctant to admit venereology patients and special Lock Hospitals, often poorly funded and staffed, offered containment (if little in the way of treatment) outside the mainstream system. The outlines of the modern system were established by the Public Health (VD) Regulations of 1916 based on the Report of the Royal Commission on Venereal Diseases (CD 8189, 1916), which recommended better facilities for diagnosis, the provision of local outpatient-based treatment centres, and the provision of free medication (invented in 1910). Patient confidentiality was an important feature of the new services for obvious reasons of patient stigma, and has remained a strong part of the culture of the specialty.

The centres had some success in reducing the levels of venereal disease within the population, but were underfinanced and remained unattractive as a career option for medical staff. In the late 1930s a Ministry of Health survey (cited by Davenport-Hines 1990: 250) found that of 357 medical officers in their 188 centres, only 63 were venereal disease specialists. The remainder professed other branches of medicine, reflecting the very low status accorded the title by their peers.

However, despite its low status, venereology, like infectious diseases, remained a relatively important acute medical specialty, requiring considerable hospital resources until the advent of penicillin and other antibiotics in the 1950s. These reduced the need for inpatient treatment to almost zero and the service rapidly became an outpatient-based, almost conveyor belt, specialty, with access to few beds and poorly developed links with the rest of the health care system.

Thus the 1960s and 1970s may be seen as a period during which three of the medical specialties that were later to play a key role in the development of services for HIV/AIDS – public health, infectious diseases, and genitourinary medicine – became marginalized, at least partly as a consequence of the perceived conquest of epidemic and infectious disease. In contrast, many acute sector specialties, such as surgery or general medicine, had been boosted by the new interventions made possible by the technological advances of the postwar years.

There were some new opportunities. Health promotion issues were beginning to be apparent in the 1970s: for instance, Cmnd 7615 (1979) recommended an expansion of health education services and of screening. Some community physicians were enthusiastic about this new focus, but others in public health who had worked with local authorities found it difficult to reframe their interests and competencies away from managing day-to-day issues to do with such matters as childhood immunization and environmental health to accommodate these more long-term aims.

A number of infectious diseases departments, faced with the decline in 'home-grown' infections, had extended their remit to include tropical medicine, which, with increasing travel to exotic locations, was becoming something of a growth industry. None the less, the specialty was not a prominent one and did not attract large resources, and the influence of many departments was diminished by their location in the old fever hospitals some distance away from the new district general hospitals.

In genitourinary medicine, however, there was less opportunity for diversification and, despite the large increase in the incidence of sexually transmitted diseases during the 1970s, concern about increasing venereal disease did not reach the formal policy agenda (unlike the anxiety about the growth of heroin addiction). Facilities were desperately inadequate throughout the country. In the late 1970s, half the 189 genitourinary medicine clinics in England and Wales were open for ten hours or less each week; some health authorities provided no service at all, while some doctors in the clinics were using inappropriate approaches to diagnosis and treatment (Adler et al. 1978).

The relative marginality of the other two clinical specialties connected with HIV/AIDS – drugs services and haemophilia – was attributable to different causes. For haemophilia the reason was simple – it was, and always had been, a small specialty because haemophilia is a rare disease. Historically a diagnosis of haemophilia, a lack of clotting factor in the blood, heralded a lifetime of pain, crippled joints and often an untimely death. There was little that medicine could do for these patients, other than to advise families against having children. During the 1970s, however, the lives of haemophiliacs were transformed when it became possible to extract the clotting factor (Factor VIII) from donated blood and inject it to control persistent bleeding. With effective treatment on offer, specialist services for haemophilia were built up and a number of localities made successful bids for so called designated 'reference centre' status, giving them a supraregional role and higher status than regional haemophilia centres. Apart from links with orthopaedics (joint disease as a result of bleeds is a common complication of haemophilia), the specialty could be seen as self-contained, and perhaps even inward-looking in nature, with a small and finite number of patients frequently known and cared for from birth throughout their lives. Haemophilia centres would often treat their patients for all their illnesses almost like a family doctor service. The Factor VIII treatment was simple and effective, and even the top specialist reference centres were run by relatively small teams of staff.

Drugs services, on the other hand, have had a more complicated history, with their evolution being marked by ideological dissensus and a pattern of historical oscillation. Policies are discarded only to be re-embraced. Crises emerge and then fade away. As Edwards (1981: 11) puts it, this evolution:

... is not just about the events of the last years or recent decades, but a story which must be seen in its rootedness. It is a story of ebb and flow in the prevalence of drugs problems, and changes in the nature of perception. Long periods of quiescence have been followed by periods of rapid transition.

In 1926 the Rolleston Committee (Ministry of Health 1926) laid down important policy guidelines when it ruled that it was acceptable practice to maintain an addict on drugs if otherwise the patient could not function satisfactorily. This relatively benign illness-based, rather than control-based, model perhaps reflected the fact that the British addict population was thought to be small and, if anything, decreasing. However, in the mid-1960s, there was increasing public and media concern about the rise in newly notified heroin addicts. A black market was now apparent on the streets and the fear of organized criminal activity grew. A drugs 'crisis' bubbled up at policy level and a series of reports and pieces of legislation followed between 1965 and 1971, with new 'drug treatment centres' run by multidisciplinary teams of medical staff and social workers set up in 1968. Berridge and Edwards (1981: 255), suggest that the covert function of the new centres was to act as containment rather than treatment centres, given the over-riding desire to contain the black market for drugs and remove addicts from criminal activity. However, this 'warehousing' role would almost certainly have been rejected by the centres themselves, many of which described themselves as 'therapeutic communities', emphasizing a psychodynamic approach to therapy and making long-term maintenance prescribing available.

Unfortunately, this new approach was no more effective than previous ones and, in the 1970s and early 1980s, some drug clinics became 'silted up' with long-term addicts on maintenance prescriptions. The result was that new places could not be offered and waiting lists grew, especially after the new heroin wave of 1979–81. Psychiatrists became very disillusioned and many reduced their involvement, as indicated by this comment from one of our research sites:

A lot of the psychiatrists here got their fingers burned to some extent being involved with drug abuse in the sixties... they became involved in that period in attempts to intervene, you know, counselling and prescribing, and found it a very unrewarding experience, and I think there was a revulsion from that really.

In some localities there was a move to a new abstinence-orientated approach to break this log jam. Addicts were asked to go through a fairly short and aggressive reduction and withdrawal programme: the phrase 'getting them through the detox' encapsulated this model. Although this may well work with well motivated addicts, the danger was that others would lose contact with formal services and have recourse to the black market.

Thus drugs services had moved from a permissive attitude to prescribing in the 1960s to an approach based on requiring total abstinence in the 1970s. Neither approach had proved generally effective, and addiction came to be seen by many as an intractable problem, while drug users themselves were perceived as very difficult and demanding patients. By the time that HIV/AIDS raised the profile of drugs services once more, many NHS-based psychiatric services offered no specialist input to drug users at all.

One thing that seems extraordinary, in retrospect, is the strength of the belief that infectious diseases had been conquered, for it was during the 1970s that hepatitis B, now known to be caused by an infectious virus transmitted (as was HIV to be a decade later) through interchange of bodily fluids, was recognized to have reached pandemic proportions. Since it could be acquired through sexual relationships, from transfused blood and blood products and from sharing needles to inject drugs, it affected patients in all the marginalized specialties described (genitourinary medicine, haemophilia and drugs services), and it was a hazard to public health. Despite this, it did not trigger sufficient concern to reach national or even local policy agendas, as recalled by a public health physician in one of our health authorities:

> We'd done a study of Hep B, and we'd found there was a real epidemic of it going on . . . and I looked at the possibility of vaccinating people, you know, susceptible groups, but everybody said 'You must be crackers . . .', so it was laughed out.

Arguably, hepatitis B could have provided, prior to HIV/AIDS, the issue to revitalize all these marginalized specialties. That it did not happen that way was, according to Muraskin (1993) a lost opportunity of tragic proportions. Instead, through processes to be described in succeeding chapters, it required the threat not just of ill-health, but death for large numbers of people, to overcome three decades of complacency about infectious diseases and to mobilize resources.

Social services

While the medical specialties that were destined to be key service providers for HIV/AIDS can be characterized as somewhat isolated and marginalized prior to the 1980s, social services, as the other professionalized organization potentially affected by the HIV/AIDS issue, had a set of different problems. In contrast to the trends towards segmentation apparent in medicine and commented on by Bucher and Strauss (1961), social work had, since 1970, been following the opposite course and pursuing greater organizational cohesion.

Social work undertaken on a voluntary basis has as long a history as medicine, but formal statutory social work organizations only began in the 1940s and it was not until 1970, following the Seebohm report (1968) that services for all the different client groups were combined into single social work departments in each local authority. Two consequences of this new arrangement were to have adverse implications for the involvement of social workers in the HIV/AIDS issue. First, it separated social work from the health service, and second, while simplifying the administrative structure, it provoked a managerial revolution in which many professional social workers seized the opportunity to become part of a 'spreading bureaucratic elite of "corporate planners" and "development executives"'. (Pearson 1978), thus greatly reducing the numbers of staff engaged in actually dealing with clients.

As all social work funding now came through the local authority, it became a complicated process to acquire social work support for medical problems such as HIV. A respondent from one of the case study sites commented: '[The consultant] actually made a bid for the support three years previously, it had taken that long to negotiate it with the social services department.'

Initially, HIV/AIDS was seen as primarily a medical problem, hence the early funding went to the health service and it was not until 1989 that specific monies were made available to local authorities. The result was that, although individual social workers were often included on early *ad hoc* committees started in key service settings within the health service, most social services departments (in any case very short of cash during the early 1980s) were comparatively late in making a strategic and policy response to the issue.

Health promotion
Health promotion is another professionalized group that has been particularly important to the development of a response to HIV/AIDS. Health promotion/education has clear content links with public health medicine, but health promotion departments are often physically separate from public health and may have considerable autonomy in how they define and organize their work. This can sometimes lead to a degree of duplication of effort, one health promotion officer, responding to our questions, said: 'Sometimes community medicine would do things that we thought we were doing, and actually if we'd known what the other was doing, between us we'd probably have done better altogether.' Health promotion officers are frequently recruited from outside the health service, often having a background in education. Like social work, health promotion has its origins long before the welfare state, and can be traced back to early concerns about the poor health of the 'working classes' and the perceived need to educate them about achieving proper standards of hygiene and

good eating habits (Lussier 1984). Interestingly, in the context of HIV/
AIDS, sexual health, and in particular contraception, was a pioneering
concern in the early years of this century, with people like Marie Stopes,
though they would not have described themselves in present-day terms as
health promotion officers, clearly acting in this role.

Over the years, with changing patterns of morbidity and mortality, there
has been a gradual change in focus in health promotion away from concerns
with disease coming from 'outside' to a greater emphasis on the effect of
an individual's behaviour on their own state of health. This approach has
been criticized for ignoring the effect of social and economic factors, which
may adversely affect people's ability to choose a 'healthy lifestyle' for
themselves (Gabbay 1992). Nevertheless, given the perceived reduction in
the importance of infectious diseases during the 1950s and 1960s, the
adoption of this approach increased the profile of health promotion during
the 1970s and 1980s.

However, as with public health, despite the rhetoric, all the evidence
suggests that on the whole prevention is accorded a lower priority, and
those working in the field a lower status, than that afforded to acute sector
treatment-orientated medicine. This holds true even when the cause of an
illness has been identified and the means of preventing it determined. For
example, as noted earlier, there has been very restricted access to hepatitis
B vaccine. Indeed, historical evidence suggests that initiatives in public
health have always been crisis-led (Bryder 1990), with interest waning as
the sense of urgency fades.

The advent of HIV/AIDS brought a strong initial emphasis on the need
for a health education offensive, with £20 million being allocated for a
nation-wide prevention campaign. In addition, low prevalence as well as
high prevalence health authorities have been encouraged to employ HIV
prevention coordinators. This has not always been seen as wholly successful, partly because having 'prevention' in their titles may well deny the
postholder access to key treatment and care sites within which much useful
preventative work may be done (Bennett 1993) and also because it may be
seen as a something of a political issue if, as often happened, they were
based within health promotion departments:

> I have never had a worker employed to work on just one issue, and
> yet I can get the money for AIDS. So it creates a fairly sensitive
> imbalance, because these posts are normally being quoted as nines
> [on the health authority pay scale]. Now in my department every-
> one's on a lesser scale . . . it created quite a few anomalies around the
> place.
>
> (district health promotion officer respondent)

Such concerns have been one factor influencing recent moves to
'embed' HIV/AIDS within other issues to do with sexual health, which the

government White Paper, *Health of the Nation* (Cm 1523 (1991)) has now endorsed. There may, however, be concerns that, in so doing, the visibility of HIV/AIDS as a health promotion issue will be reduced.

Pre-existing voluntary sector settings

As we shall see, it was the voluntary groups arising from social movements connected with the gay community that were to have the most telling influence on service development, and these particular organizations only arose in response to HIV/AIDS. However, there had been an upsurge in voluntarism in the postwar period[2] and a number of pre-existing voluntary organizations moved into this new field. Some were already working in spheres, such as drugs services and haemophilia, on which HIV/AIDS made a specific and direct impact, others were drawn from a range of social welfare fields, such as the Church of England's Boards for Social Responsibility, the Salvation Army and Barnardo's.

The different organizations may perhaps be seen as representing different points on a continuum between the conflict and consensus traditions of voluntary action, before arriving at the true social movement organizations represented by those arising from the gay movement, which we discuss in the next section.

Closest to consensus come the various religious groups and organizations involved in childcare. These may be said to represent the views of what might be termed the liberal end of the 'moral majority'. In particular various organizations run by, or originally associated with, the churches have been prominent here, confirming the continuation into the modern day of the traditional involvement of religious organizations with the provision of welfare (Rooff 1957). For many of these, HIV meant extending their remit only slightly. There were already organizations working with such groups as prostitutes, drug users, women and children in need, homeless people and the dying, it needed little imagination to see that HIV/AIDS was just one more problem to add to the many these groups were already experiencing. In addition, before long it became clear that, for once, a welfare issue looked likely to be capable of attracting large amounts of funding, and organizations were not slow in recognizing the utility of making the HIV connection: 'I am under no illusion, we wouldn't have got [the project] off the ground nearly so quickly if it hadn't been for the fact that we *could* [respondent's emphasis] be helping women who were HIV positive' (voluntary sector respondent).

Voluntary drugs services in particular have had a long history, especially in the provision of residential care. Some were, or had been, associated with religious organizations, but others, as noted earlier, had often been closely associated with the statutory sector. In many cases they had experienced a similar history to the statutory drugs services, with the idealistic and permissive 'therapeutic communities' of the 1950s and 1960s changing, if they survived the ensuing chaos, into institutions reflecting the hardline approach favoured by drug abuse services in the statutory sector during the 1970s and early 1980s. However, just prior to the recognition that injecting drug users were at risk from HIV/AIDS, the focus had moved away from medical intervention to encouraging the involvement of voluntary organizations. The Advisory Council on the Misuse of Drugs (ACMD), in its 1982 report had advised that community-based services were often more accessible and attractive to drug misusers than those the statutory services had been offering. In response, in 1983 the Department of Health, set up a central funding initiative and invited applications for funding local community projects on the problem of drug abuse.

When the HIV/AIDS issue arose, it was often such new projects that were small enough and flexible enough to respond positively to the sudden change of emphasis from promoting abstinence to providing clean injecting equipment within a new policy of harm reduction, where older, more established organizations found it difficult to accommodate the new approach.

In contrast to drugs services, provided by volunteers *for* drug users, the Haemophilia Society was a self-help organization run by those directly affected by the disease, either themselves, or as relatives of people with haemophilia. At national level, the organization was formally constituted and employed paid staff, but there were also numerous small local organizations, which varied in how active they were at any one time. These groups, too were often initiated and/or serviced by professional staff in the haemophilia centres.

By no means all people with haemophilia belonged to one of these groups, and they often focused more on the needs of parents, particularly mothers of young haemophiliac boys, than on providing services for adults who, following the advent of Factor VIII were encouraged to play down their illness and 'get on with their lives' in as normal a way as possible.

Not that Factor VIII was the total panacea, as it was accepted that, as each dose represented several pints of transfused blood, it was highly likely to be contaminated with any blood-borne viral infection currently going the rounds. During the 1970s, that meant hepatitis B, particularly if the supply came from the USA where commercial blood banks made a habit of targeting the gay community as an easily identified and readily accessible source of donors (Sapolsky and Boswell 1992). Long before the even worse problem of HIV was recognized, some doctors in Britain were concerned about the heavy viral contamination in the US Factor VIII and took action to restrict its use where possible: 'We had the view that NHS material was probably safer . . . just had a general gut feeling, made a policy . . . of preserving as far as possible NHS material for children.'

This far-sighted policy ultimately meant that almost all the children attending that haemophilia centre were found to be free of HIV when tests became available, in contrast to some other centres where a large proportion had acquired the virus.

This raises the question of how issues rise up the agenda, even in voluntary organizations supposedly focused on the welfare of their members. It might have been thought that the Haemophilia Society would have been in a position to lobby long before HIV for the provision of an adequate supply of uncontaminated Factor VIII. Why did they not do so, or at any rate, not effectively? Since tragedy struck and the enormity of their position was recognized there has been massive lobbying, not only for compensation, but for the provision of Factor VIII of exceptional purity. One answer may be suggested by Klandermans' (1992) observation that the roots of social protest lie in interpretations, not reality, and that it is from the reconstruction of the situation that new actions emerge. In the 1970s, as we noted earlier, infections were treated as of little importance by medical professionals and the general public alike. It is only now, when AIDS has forced the reinterpretation of the situation, that lack of adequate control of cross-infection has become something to protest about. Thus the Haemophilia Society should perhaps be seen as a voluntary organization now moving closer to the conflict end of the continuum than in its previous existence prior to HIV/AIDS.

Social movement organization-based settings

Social movements are related to consciousness of oppression (discrimination in relation to class, race, etc.), which may have a very long history indeed. However, identifiable social movements tend to have shorter histories, with cycles of protest (Tarrow 1983) rising and falling, and the SMOs, which are their structural manifestation, may have shorter histories still. Not only are they subject to cyclical waxing and waning of interest in the cause, but to organizational lifecycle factors in which a drift towards institutionalization (Lohdahl and Mitchell 1980) may erode original ideals and objectives.

As will be discussed at greater length in Chapter 4, a number of quite separate social movements with their roots in the 1960s and 1970s, such as consumerism, 'alternative' medicine, the hospice movement, community care and, most importantly, gay liberation, have contributed to the development of the SMOs, which have since become, in the words of Patton (1990) the 'AIDS Service Industry'. However, most of the SMOs themselves date only from the early 1980s, and were either formed in response to the appearance of HIV/AIDS, or, if already existing in some form (as for instance with the Shanti project in San Francisco, which was originally for people dying of cancer), were totally taken over and transformed by their new role.

The early AIDS service organizations were in many ways archetypal SMOs, with their immediate roots in a radical gay activist culture. There is a general debate about how effective SMOs are in intervening in formal decision-making processes. Some theorists of social movements have seen them as sectarian and backward-looking, unable to play a role in advanced societies (Touraine 1981). This suggests that the interface between a radical voluntary sector and a more ostensibly value neutral public sector bureaucracy (at least in the way that it represents itself to the world) may be difficult to cross. The more value-laden the SMO, the more it may approximate to the sect where there is strong exclusivity (Wilson 1967), or even withdrawal from the secular world, thus making it less effective as a change agent except within its own narrow confines.

There can be little doubt that a particular set of values coming from existing gay organizations strongly affected the policies and approaches of early AIDS service organizations. Padgug and Oppenheimer (1992) point out:

> The community has, through its political and legal structures . . . insisted that the gay community has the right to determine whether specific public health and related measures proposed as weapons in the fight against AIDS . . . will have adverse or positive effects on its civil rights or liberties.

Nevertheless, neither such non-mainstream attitudes, nor the low profile of the issue in the early years, prevented these early organizations from quickly making a very considerable impact on government officials and policy makers. Within eighteen months of its birth in 1982, for example, Gay Men's Health Crisis in New York was presenting documentation on the issue to the United States Conference of Mayors and was beginning to attract government funding (Perrow and Guillen 1990). Perhaps, as Padgug and Oppenheimer (1992) suggest, a 'lack of other claimants to the ownership of AIDS', made their involvement more acceptable than it would otherwise have been. Whatever the reasons, the history of SMOs in relation to the AIDS issue, as Arno's (1986) case study of service developments in San Francisco illustrates, suggests that in certain circumstances such groupings can work well within more formal decision-making systems.

The first organization to be formed specifically for HIV/AIDS in Britain, the London-based Terrence Higgins Trust (THT) was, like its US counterparts, also founded by gay men. However, Watney (1988) sees it as having had a different cultural background: 'British gay culture is fragmentary and atomised, lacking even the most elementary civil rights consciousness, unable even to organize a proper national newspaper.' Watney attributes this to the repressive effect of 'centuries of British homophobia'. Despite this, the history of THT as described by Schramm-Evans (1990) does not look so different from that of similar groups in other countries, which Watney sees as less hostile. From an initial core group formed in 1983, funded entirely through the gay community, by 1985 its lobbying activities had gained it sufficient credibility within government circles for it to receive a grant of £35,000, a fair achievement for an organization arising from such an apparently unpromising situation.

THT and its prototype, the Gay Men's Health Crisis in New York, became models for all the other gay-initiated AIDS Service Organizations, which appeared in almost every major city, demonstrating the efficacy of the gay communications network even where the community was seen as less organized. In all our early responding provincial health authorities, for example, THT lookalikes were established within a few months of the initial publicity about the London organization. This account, taken from the first newsletter issued by one such organization, was typical of those we encountered:

> I attended a gathering of people interested in doing something positive to fight the disease AIDS. The first meeting was held in the [club] on Sunday afternoon in December 1984.

> I knew that after listening to Tony Whitehead from the Terrence Higgins Trust that I was able to offer my services to help with forming a Committee and in fund raising.

> I took the names and addresses of various people and organizations interested in helping. Another meeting was held in the [club] on Sunday 3rd March 1985 . . . [and] I found myself appointed Secretary . . . The committee at the time consisted of seven people.

However, while such an account might be seen as representative of the startup phase of any small voluntary organization, these were very different organizations from most of those that the statutory sector was used to dealing with. Their membership were neither willing to act as an uncritical voluntary labourforce, told what to do by those nominally 'in charge'; nor did they wish to act unilaterally as autonomous organizations. Instead they saw themselves as having a key role to play within the statutory sector, in preventative activity, in service planning and delivery and in developing policy, and they demanded collaboration and involvement in a quite unprecedented way.

The speed and degree to which they succeeded in these aims depended greatly on local social and political factors. In some localities opposition to the gay movement in general was entrenched, and nascent AIDS service organizations took some time to get established. In other places with a more radical social and political tradition, and where key people in the statutory sector offered support, they quickly gained what was to some opponents a rather disconcerting degree of credibility. Indeed in Britain, as we shall see later, people originating from SMOs have had some success in capturing the specialist HIV labour market set up within the NHS after official funding became available.

The widespread presence of SMOs or of social movement insurgency within formal public sector organizations poses a dilemma. On the one hand, this can lead to intense energy, commitment and a stress on basic affirmative values. Downs (1967) argues that organizations operating in complex and changing environments in fact need 'zealots' to break up the received wisdom. Such staff may, in effect, be acting as 'bureaucratic insurgents' (Zald and Berger 1978) from within:

> Early on I had quite a major row with Dr X . . . about what coun-selling was and how medics were not providing this; and he was dreadfully upset, not just because of the content of the counselling but because of the status of the medical and voluntary sectors . . . I don't think he grasped that at that stage the voluntary sector was leading the way.

Outcomes of such insurgency are identified by Zald and Berger (1978) as either failure and repression, or varying degrees of organizational tol-eration or incorporation. The AIDS service organizations were fortunate in that public perception of the importance and relevance of the issue they were promoting – HIV/AIDS – changed. Even those organizations that were relatively unsuccessful during the prelegitimation phase became re-spectable and improved links with the statutory sector once the issue gained government support, and those that had become established early, par-ticularly the Terrence Higgins Trust, came to be seen as expert in the field and exerted tremendous influence on policy at the highest level.

This legitimation and incorporation into statutory sector systems can be seen both as a major strength of the AIDS service organizations and a crucial weakness. A strength in that their views were an important influ-ence on the character of service development for HIV/AIDS; a weakness, because in consequence they became dependent on the high levels of government funding they attracted, leading to power shifting to a paid salariat (Freeman 1992) and away from their original roots in voluntarism and activism. The picture that is now beginning to emerge of the devel-opment over time of these AIDS service organizations is well described in Patton (1990: Chapter 1) and Schramm-Evans' (1990) case analysis of THT provides a perfect example. Schramm-Evans notes THT's fluid and creative early phase, its explosive growth, escalating administrative problems, its increasing dependence on government funding, its retreat from radical ideology and the emergence of an internal bureaucracy. Interestingly, there has been a recent emergence of new organizations such as ACT UP (AIDS Coalition to Unleash Power), formed to reradicalize the voluntary sector approach to HIV/AIDS following the perceived bureaucratization and professionalization of the earlier organizations (Padgug and Oppenheimer

1992). As, in social movement terms, there is nothing to indicate that the voluntary sector response to the issue has waned, this suggests that the influence of such universal organizational processes as lifecycles, noted earlier, may be stronger than the context in which they arise.

However, it must also be recalled some of those who took an early lead in development were themselves HIV infected and have since become ill or died, raising an issue about ensuring continuity of leadership. Although there is disagreement among authors over the precise effect of leadership succession on organizational performance (Allen et al. 1979), most seem agreed that it does make a difference. Self-help organizations such as Body Positive, where membership is entirely drawn from those infected, are particularly at risk and one early organization, Frontliners (people with an AIDS diagnosis), was unable to sustain itself and has folded. In broader management terms, Beatty and Zajac (1987) specifically identify unexpected changes of leadership as likely to be perceived as destabilizing, leading to outside investors withdrawing support, and our research suggests that such perceptions may be one factor in the observed reluctance of many statutory organizations to give financial support to the voluntary sector.

Concluding remarks

In this chapter, we have tried to analyse the characteristics of a number of key service settings that were engaged in shaping the early response to HIV/AIDS. The notion of a 'setting' (Sarason 1976) was indeed seen as helpful as sensitizing us to how it was that services developed at local level.

The first general point that emerges is that the emergent HIV/AIDS field was characterized by an exceptionally high degree of inter- and intra-organizational complexity. Within the health care sector alone, a number of specialties were involved, each with its own history, model of care and way of working. Moreover, social care and SMO-based settings were also important deliverers of service outside the health service. Most of these settings, however, could be seen at least initially as relatively powerless and marginal given the preoccupation with acute medicine. Not only were a number of different organizations involved, but more abstractly also a number of different types of organizations.

The response from each segment was heavily shaped by its own history and established identity. This historic context could involve important moral, social and political components as well as medical issues. So, for instance, drugs services had a unique relationship with a central bureaucracy of control, while haemophilia, traditionally an inward-looking specialty, perhaps found it difficult to adapt to working across boundaries.

However, the HIV/AIDS epidemic provoked change as well as signalling continuity within these settings. For instance, while at one level they were heavily influenced by their past, genitourinary medicine services have also developed rapidly throughout the 1980s (Monks Report, Department of Health 1988), with a new infrastructure and a new generation of consultants moving into post. Many of these settings, previously searching for a *raison d'être*, were energized by the HIV epidemic. This presents a rather different picture from the strong routinization and lifecycle effects suggested by Sarason (1976). Perhaps existing settings were propelled into a new organizational lifecycle with the stimulus of HIV/AIDS?

The three blocs identified by Alford (1975) were all present in the HIV/AIDS field. However SMOs could not be seen as representing a repressed 'community' interest but were far more proactive than in his model. As we shall see later, SMOs were increasingly able to use public funding to build up a considerable degree of 'free space' and develop significant service systems outside the 'official' sector. There is a paucity of research (except for Zald and Berger 1978) that addresses organization theory from a social movement perspective. However, Soeters (1986), in his reanalysis of Peters and Waterman's (1982) 'excellent companies' as SMOs essentially characterized by strong collective cultures, suggests that this is an area worthy of further development. This argument is confirmed by our study of service development in the HIV/AIDS field.

Notes

1 For example public health, now one of the pillars of establishment medicine, was a new and radical issue in the Victorian era, and social services also had its roots in numerous campaigning movements of that period.
2 Sainsbury (1977) notes that, in 1970, there were 76,648 charitable organizations listed with the charity commissioners, and that 10,000 of these had been registered within the last ten years.

HIV/AIDS – the influence of ideologies

HAROLD BRIDGES LIBRARY
S. MARTIN'S COLLEGE
LANCASTER

Introduction

We now turn from looking at particular settings to consider more generally how ideologies, sets of subjective beliefs, values and meanings (Snow and Benford 1992), helped to shape the response to HIV/AIDS at personal, organizational and societal levels. The part ideologies have played in this process is theoretically interesting because mainstream organizational theory has been weak in analysing the relationship between changes in society, societally situated ideologies and the particular organization under study. Consider such questions as:

- How is it possible to develop drugs services in a community where there is a strong value system that operates to condemn any form of drug use?
- Why is it possible to make a compulsory detention order in relation to someone with HIV, and why should this meet with resistance from some?
- Why are alternative health care systems, such as homeopathy, healing through crystals or aromatherapy, so prevalent in the field of HIV/ AIDS?

Such questions direct us to consider the role of values and beliefs in mediating actions, and in so doing to broaden the debate about the role of subjective rather than objective thought, the unconscious rather than the conscious, in shaping action within organizations.

The concept of ideology has similarities with that of 'organizational culture' so popular in the 1980s but takes it in both a more conflictual and more societally embedded direction. For instance, writers such as Schein (1985) have taken a very plastic and top down view of organizational culture: 'The further I got into the topic of organizational culture, the more I realized that culture was the result of entrepreneurial activities by company founders, leaders of movements, institution builders and social architects.'

By contrast, we argue that in the HIV/AIDS field, while development of a new organizational culture has been of central importance in determining the response to such an unusual epidemic, this emerging consciousness was clearly associated with the longer term and collective growth of various social movements. Consciousness arose more than being shaped. Thus health care organizations had to be seen as profoundly embedded in their historical and societal context and much less amenable to transformational leadership from the top or to 'culture busting' than much of the literature of the 1980s implied (see Pettigrew and Whipp (1991) for a similar discussion in relation to managing strategic change in the private sector).

We also need to explore the concept of 'ideology' itself in greater detail. We argue that it should not be understood solely in ethnomethodological terms of symbolism, language and meaning but also in political science terms of supplying formal propositions – a doctrinal orthodoxy – which structures reality, supplies stereotypes of other social groupings and leads to a set of actions. Perhaps the term ideology equates, at a more concrete level of analysis, with the concept of a 'mind set', a set of ideas about a particular issue that may be shaped by, but is not identical to, a person's general ideological stance towards more global themes.

While we focus on the specific case of service development for HIV/AIDS, these issues are much more general. There has been much work on other aspects of cognition within organizations, for example, the role of 'organizational sagas' in defining a collective folk memory (Clark 1972), yet the role of ideology is often treated within such literature with a broad brush. However, the term 'ideology' surely implies more systemic, internally consistent, and action-orientated attributes than these other conceptions of 'myths', 'sagas' or 'culture'.

In this chapter we first look at the concept of ideology, and consider its relevance to organization theory. We then move on to consider and illustrate with empirical examples – first, four very different perspectives of the epidemic based on the dominant ideologies of four policy constituencies, and second, some key general areas in which we see ideologies and mindsets as having influenced the direction of service development for HIV/AIDS. Finally, we consider to what extent these findings are specific to the HIV/AIDS issue, or are generic processes that are potentially generalizable to other organizational issues both within the NHS and outside it.

Ideology, energy and change

'Ideology' represents a vast and complex field within social science, and we can do little more here than touch upon some of the key debates. A good recent overview of the current status of the field is supplied by Boudon (1989), who takes an overview of the development of various definitions of ideology and rehearses a range of current thinking on the subject.

Going back to the beginning he suggests that for Marx, the term 'ideology' held a negative concept, as he saw ideologies as essentially false ideas that social actors possessed because of their 'material interaction'. Lenin, on the other hand, saw ideology much more functionally as an ideas system used by protagonists in social struggles (here the class struggle). It is in this sense that the term is often used today, reflecting the interest theory of ideology, in which different work groups may be seen as adopting ideologies that benefit their own economic interests. Non-Marxist sociologists have also worked in this area, going back to Pareto's concept of 'derivations', which are seen as intellectual constructs that people devise to show that their feelings are justified. More recently, Aron (1977) drew attention to the way in which political ideologies mixed together both descriptive and prescriptive elements, alerting us to the rhetorical devices employed by the ideologue:

> Political ideologies always combine, more or less felicitously, factual propositions and value judgements. They express an outlook on the world and a will turned towards the future. They do not fall directly under the choice of true or false nor do they belong to the same category as taste or colour.

Shils (1968) similarly highlighted some of the negative and zealous features of ideological thought systems: their rejection of innovation, the intolerant nature of their precepts, the affective way in which they are promulgated, the adherence they demand and their association with institutional enforcement mechanisms.

Such generally negative concepts of 'ideology' are shared by Boudon, whose general thesis is based on a definition of ideology as inevitably based on 'false or dubious ideas'. This position is, in our view, debatable, and in any case does not assist us in understanding the processes by which beliefs and values, whether or not these are based on some basic 'truth', influence processes of change within society. Geertz (1973), however, does address this question. Geertz was not so interested in the traditional question of whether ideologies were true or false so much as in how ideology could arise as a response to uncertainty and strain, providing a much needed guide for action and source of mobilization. Thus, within a ethnomethodological perspective, Geertz stresses the role of symbols, tropes and metaphors, rather than formal propositions, in defining ideological thought, which should be seen above all as a source of symbolic action. In particular it provides a rhetorical guide for political action under conditions of uncertainty:

> Further, as the various sorts of cultural symbolism are extrinsic sources of information, templates for the organization of social and psychological processes, they come most crucially into play in situations where the particular kind of information they contain is lacking, where institutionalized guides for behaviour, thought or feeling are weak or absent. It is in country unfamiliar emotionally or topographically that one needs poems and road maps.
> (Geertz 1973: 218)

Boudon (1989) has criticized Geertz's position precisely because of an overemphasis on metaphor as a source of meaning. However, its advantage is that it directs us away from a highly negative concept of ideology, and highlights the links between the possession of ideologies and political action. For example, Hall and Jacques (1983) (following Gramsci's notion of intellectual hegemony) argue that the rise of Thatcherism in the 1980s has to be understood as an instance of a successful ideological project; while others (Jessop et al. 1984) have criticized this position for excessive emphasis on idealism. Our own position in relation to the HIV/AIDS field is, as we shall see in the succeeding sections, that the evidence suggests that ideologies did matter, with the strongest of them providing a key group resource with which to define the situation and impel to action.

Has 'ideology' been neglected within organization theory?

It is interesting that alongside a perceived emphasis on hard-nosed and performance-related studies in management research of the 1980s, an increasing number of studies have acknowledged the importance of subjective dimensions within organizations. In many cases, however, there has not been an extended discussion of the term 'ideology'. Sometimes the word 'ideology' has been used, but often loosely and with little reference to the social scientific literature available elsewhere. This weakness was pointed out as early as Starbuck (1982). Nevertheless, though maybe not overtly acknowledged as such, we would argue that the concept of ideology has clearly been influential in extending understanding of organizational processes in recent years.

Initially, recognition of the influence of beliefs and values on organizational behaviour came along with the reaction against the purely quantitative approach to organizational dimensions (characteristic of the Aston School's work of the 1960s), and began as early as the 1970s. Pettigrew's (1973a) study of the pattern of relations between different subunits in a retailing firm, for example, focused on decision-making as a political process rather than as determined by measures of organizational structure. Alongside different relationships to the pattern of work, these groups typically displayed different values or beliefs (or even stereotypes about each other) that made decision-making more conflictual. However, such beliefs perhaps could be seen as useful tools in a power struggle rather than as an end in themselves (Beyer 1981). Certainly these beliefs were less intense, complex and coherent than the notion of 'ideology' might imply.

The question of values could be even more important in certain charged organizational contexts. Beyer's (1981: 166) review, for instance, argued that a group of normatively based organizations (such as churches, political parties and SMOs) may attract and retain members on the basis of particular ideologies. Within such organizations:

> The ideology mobilizes consciousness and action by connecting social burdens with general ethical principles. The result is that commitment is provided to perform everyday organizational tasks on the way to some grand scheme of things.
>
> (Beyer 1981: 166)

Here we see the beginnings of the idea that an ideology may provide the high commitment needed to provide energy for long-term change. However, while Beyer reviews macro level national cultures as sources of ideologies and values, and also micro level individual organizations and roles, she does not consider the more specific question of how change within certain sectors of society may become a source of new ideologies.

Brunsson's (1982) study of decision-making processes in seven private and public sector organizations looked at the role of organizational ideologies in simplifying the decision-making process. Unlike Boudon and many other writers on ideology, Brunnson does not attempt to make value judgements on 'truth' or 'falsity' but simply defines 'ideology' as a 'set of ideas', distinguishing between individual cognitive structures ('subjective ideology'), members' ideas of the cognitive structures of their colleagues ('perceived ideologies') and ideas shared by all organizational members affording common bases for discussion and action ('objective ideologies'). This approach seems to offer a potentially fruitful frame for understanding the role of beliefs and values in mediating action. Unfortunately, however, Brunnson did not really explore the question of how ideologies arise, how conflict between different ideologies presents in the same organization or whether ideologies are organizationally specific or more widely societally embedded.

Meyer's (1982) study of two hospitals in crisis suggested that coherent 'ideologies' (here seen in Geertz-like terms of the beliefs, stories and language systems generated from the particular administrative subculture) can supplant formal structures as effective shapers of responses to environmental disturbances. This is clearly relevant to processes evident in the response to HIV/AIDS, but again, ideology was seen as organizationally specific and ideological conflicts between different segments within the hospitals were not studied.

Meyer suggested that ideologies exert strong forces in guiding organizational responses to unanticipated events in the environment, with the advantages that they engender devotion, lend drama and accord dignity to everyday activities. During crises, they can shape responses and provide reservoirs of goodwill that sanction unusual responses. However, Meyer also recognized that potent ideologies can also cause organizations to become excessively deviant, rigid and stagnant, and indeed members of such organizations may suffer from distorted perceptions of the outside world.

Johnson (1990), in his useful review of recent developments in the strategic change literature, notes first of all the retreat from long-range, formalistic approaches to strategic management, and a move towards seeing organizations as containing important social, political and cognitive elements. Johnson refers very broadly to core beliefs and assumptions that operate within an organization, including myths, language, ceremonies, interpretive schemas, dominant logics or paradigms, all of which structure organizational reality, and suggest that the achievement of radical strategic change is unlikely without parallel changes to these underlying cognitive schemas.

While Johnson sensitizes us to the importance of subjective aspects of organizational reality, the concept of 'ideology' – although referred to – needs to be explored rather further. Moreover, this account sees organizational culture as relatively malleable by top management, at least under crisis conditions. So symbolic and political actions could be employed by purposeful change agents in questioning and breaking down the adherence to current norms and political structures and in building and signalling a 'counter-culture'. Indeed, major change processes are seen as becoming highly personalized upon a very few individual leaders.

Our data suggest, however, that in effecting change in response to HIV/AIDS deliberate use of such techniques by identifiable change agents was rare (though there were occasional exceptions), and that the contribution of ideology to mediating change had to be seen as much more diffuse, intangible, and, indeed, developmental. We would thus argue that, while organization theory has clearly moved towards more openness to addressing subjective as well as objective processes, it may still need further elaboration in its treatment of ideology. All too often it is assumed that cultural or ideological change can be understood within the context of the single organization, rather than society. The sources of ideology are not explored in depth. Notions of ideology – if explored at all – tend to the ethnomethodological, with an emphasis on language, metaphor and meaning rather than doctrine. Culture shaping is also often seen as the purposeful province of top management, rather than as a messy, unpredictable and collective endeavour.

We suggest in this chapter that 'ideology' in the context of the development of services for HIV/AIDS cannot be seen as an ephemeral, plastic and non-contested product of single organizations, as implied in some of the organization theory reviewed, but rather as a concept that is much more collective, and more historically and socially embedded. Our overall argument is that the responses made to HIV/AIDS by individuals, groups and health care organizations working in the field were influenced by a number of very different and societally embedded interpretations of the epidemic, and that these were mediated by previously constructed attitudes and values. We suggest, further, the possibility of analysing these interpretations at two levels: (1) as relatively coherent ideological perspectives, providing general frameworks through which different groups construed reality (Berger and Luckmann 1966); and (2) as 'mind sets', which more closely applied general ideologies to particular issues and preceded action. Mind sets have similarities with psychological concepts such as 'schemas' (mental structures of knowledge that we project onto evidence (Bartlett 1932)) and 'frames' (data-structures that can be adapted to fit reality by changing details as necessary (Minsky 1977)).

Kelly's (1955) personal construct theory, in which he argues that people have a complex conceptual framework that allows the ideas that are most important to them to take precedence over others that are less important, is also very relevant. It offers an explanation for some being more concerned about, say, morality than freedom, when both are conceived to be 'good' things. An example from the HIV/AIDS field would be the conflict between those who define homosexuality as immoral, and therefore to be suppressed, by legislation if necessary, and those for whom civil liberties are of primary importance.

In the next two sections we explore this idea further; first by considering some key ideologically based perspectives through which the epidemic was seen by different groups of influential players, and moving on in the next section to look more specifically at the effect of particular sets of attitudes, beliefs and values on aspects of service development.

The HIV/AIDS epidemic in four perspectives

We suggest in this section some alternative definitions of the HIV/AIDS epidemic from four different vantage points, which can in turn be dubbed: (1) conservative; (2) radical; (3) liberal; and (4) professional. Each defined its own constituency. The first interpretation might be identified among liberal intellectuals in the higher levels of public administration; the second came from those (mainly medical) people for whom (although their ranks

included protagonists of other perspectives) their professional status imposed a distinct viewpoint and value system of its own; the third emerged
from, in particular the gay movement, but also from a number of other
social movements that were gaining influence during the 1970s and early
1980s; and the fourth came from conservative and religious groups or
individuals whose leanings were towards 'old fashioned' virtues and moral
standards.

Although these ideologies coexisted, it is important to see them also in
a historical context, perhaps as part of a cyclical process of changing
values and attitudes. Thus Thatcherite conservatism, though chronologi-
cally the most recent, modelled itself explicitly on values seen as having
been those espoused by Victorian society, while liberalism and the radical
left, most visible during the 'permissive' decades of the 1960s and 1970s,
perhaps echoed other periods characterized by liberal intellectualism (e.g.
the 1920s) and by radical action.

It is also possible to see each of these four vantage points as representing
two dynamically different influences on process. In these terms, we may
see the liberal and professional perspectives as representing forces towards
either maintaining continuity or, if change was inevitable or deemed necessary, incorporating this into the fabric of society in as incremental and
non-controversial manner as possible. On the other hand, though each
would no doubt reject the idea of any kind of alliance, the campaigning
and ideological stances taken by both conservatism under Margaret Thatcher
and radical SMOs are similar in their rejection of continuity in favour of
dynamic and, if necessary, confrontational change.

The liberal mandarins: reformism from above

We start with the point of view of higher reaches of the health policy and
management process. For them, HIV/AIDS represented just another policy
issue that they had to process, albeit a controversial one that could arouse
passion in a variety of unusual quarters. Their world can be seen as having
arisen from the liberal intellectual tradition of the 1960s. It was embedded
in a tiny London-based (albeit with outposts in Oxford and Cambridge)
liberal mandarinate, which continued to make policy, sit on advisory committees, run key cultural and intellectual institutions such as the BBC or
the universities, write letters to *The Times* and in general dictate the terms
of policy debate.

The traditional or Christian right was firmly marginalized. At the BBC
of the 1960s, the moral campaigner, Mary Whitehouse, it was famously
remarked by Hugh Greene (Director General of the BBC), was not only
persona non grata but *persona non exista*. In the long tradition of the
Fabian society, single-issue pressure groups sought to influence and per-
meate this elite, rather than confront it. There were social links across

to groups of writers and intellectuals (such as the Bloomsbury Group) who themselves led freewheeling private lives. It had been long apparent that not everyone in such circles was in a monogamous heterosexual relationship.

The liberal elite's norms were strongly those of clubbability, respect for personal privacy, and civilized behaviour. They wanted to make the country a freer and happier place, and greater personal and sexual freedom was an important part of their agenda. Aware of the massive discrepancy between what was an open secret within the elite, and what could be said in public, this sense of hypocrisy perhaps led to the drive for reform, including the decriminalization of homosexuality. There was recourse to the classic device of a Committee of Enquiry, which had been staffed by 'the good and the great', such as a Vice Chancellor (Wolfenden), who could safely be left to come up with 'civilized' but not radical conclusions in due course.

This pre-Thatcherite world of the liberal metropolitan elite is well described by Annan (1991). His book, *Our Age: Portrait of a Generation*, ends with their being booed off the stage by the new Thatcherite order in 1979. These mandarins also found their world shaken by the emergence of unexpectedly radical movements to the left of them in the 1970s. They had not expected the Gay Liberation Front (GLF) at all:

> *Our Age* blinked. Who were these hard left creatures in dungarees, trumpeting *Time Out* values, sporting pink triangle badges and glowering instead of camping? Whether or not homosexuals liked it, they were now in politics.
>
> (Annan 1991: 151)

However, Annan sees the ancient pattern reasserting itself in the response of British elites to HIV/AIDS. The government, alongside royalty and the churches, is seen as compassionate and liberal. What is more, such elites could easily mobilize significant resources, both in money and symbolic terms.

Surely a touch of this mandarin sensibility is evident in Fox et al.'s (1989) interpretation of the policy response to HIV/AIDS in the USA, Britain and Sweden. This essentially argues that the pattern of decision-making carried on in its usual closed manner; diseases may come and diseases may go, but health care policy-making goes on for ever. So the main response to AIDS was seen as shaped by the technical doctrines and liberal values of elite groupings and (it could be added) higher civil service and NHS management. The liberal elite quickly established its own consensus, which defined the epidemic in such a way as to head off attempts to introduce massive control measures:

> Policy in the three countries has, in the main, been based on consensus, both professional and political: a consensus that has ruled out

certain options (like widespread mandated screening for infection) ... (and) on agreement that the epidemic, whatever its unique features and however menacing it might appear, is a disease like any other as far as research and treatment is concerned.

(Fox et al. 1989)

Ideological aspects of professionalism

The 'liberal mandarins' of the last section were ably assisted and their views reinforced by those to whom government would naturally turn for advice on the appropriate response to a new health issue, the medical profession.

Professionalism is most frequently seen by sociologists as a set of defining attributes, such as autonomy, expertise and norms of conduct (Wilensky 1964) rather than as an ideology in its own right. Nevertheless as writers such as Dibble (1962) and Freidson (1988) point out, the very construction of this coherent definitional framework requires the existence of a set of attitudes, beliefs and values to which members of professional groups must adhere in order to 'belong'. Elliott (1973), states this very simply when he says: 'The concept of professional ideology has a basis in the everyday experience that members of the same occupational group tend to think and behave in characteristic ways.'

Medicine is often cited as the archetypical example of a 'profession'. Its members are seen as, first and foremost, part of a scientific culture (Mishler 1981) and pre-eminent in their knowledge of and expertise in the field of health and illness (Freidson 1988). Doctors are highly regarded by a public that sees itself as, by and large, dependent on the profession for the technological help required to restore and maintain optimum physical (and possibly mental) function, and trusts in the perceived ideals of professional service to deliver whatever interventions are required (Parsons 1951).

As a consequence of their perceived professionalism, doctors have acquired both power and status. However, as medical technology has advanced, the delivery of health care has become increasingly costly and governments, rather than individuals, have had to intervene and regulate its provision. Freddi (1989) argues that this has inevitably had an adverse effect on the autonomy vested in the profession and that, in order to maintain some degree of this, doctors have had to become closely involved in the political process to legitimate and protect their own professional structures and operational standards.

Hence, since the beginning of the welfare state and the institution of the NHS, the medical profession, and in particular representatives of those members of the profession who work in the field of public health, have worked closely with and in government departments. There may have been some loss of autonomy, but the opportunity to influence and often determine government policy on health care has probably been seen as compensatory, at least by those privileged to walk in the corridors of power.

Thus the ideology of the profession became institutionalized within government departments dealing with health care issues and, when the issue of AIDS first arose, and government became aware of a potential health crisis to which it must respond, it was to this group of public health physicians that ministers and government officials turned for guidance. Hence this professional ideology emphasizing the controlled, non-judgemental, essentially 'scientific' approach to the problem, combined with the norms of 'civilized' behaviour held by the liberal mandarins, mediated the response to the epidemic, and the Chief Medical Officer, Sir Donald Acheson, received much praise for his handling of the issue. The approach taken is well illustrated by the heading to an article by Polly Toynbee in the *Guardian* in March 1987: 'No moralising, no politics – just a no-nonsense, medically-based campaign. This was how Sir Donald Acheson tackled the Cabinet.' Or, as Fox et al. (1989) put it, the social construction of the epidemic at government level as a professional issue meant that it was defined as mainly a problem for the experts and could be seen as 'an unseemly subject for partisan debate'.

The radicals: the gay social movement and other ideologies

We now move on to other, more radical ideological perspectives that shaped the response to HIV/AIDS. Foremost amongst these, as we have already indicated, was the gay social movement. The Wolfenden Report (CMND 247 1957), recommending the partial decriminalization of homosexuality, was the start of a political struggle to reform the law by an increasingly radical and visible gay community, epitomized by the GLF. The ten-year campaign culminated in the passing of the 1967 Sexual Offences Act legalizing homosexual acts between consenting adults in private, and although GLF did not survive for long, as Philips (1988) points out, its influence persisted long afterwards because it fitted so well with the developing social culture of the period:

> GLF appeared to catch the mood of the time perfectly: the growth of the Women's Liberation Movement and the recognition of sexism; actions taken by Black people against racism; the growth of youth culture as expressed in the anti-Vietnam demonstrations, music and clothes. I became aware that GLF was offering gay men and women the opportunity to become part of that growing radical climate as open and proud homosexuals.

However, as Padgug and Oppenheimer (1992) note, the arrival of AIDS, as well as presenting a major and unexpected physical threat to the gay community within which it was first identified, also challenged the whole ideology surrounding gay culture and the 'exuberant sexuality' with which it was associated. Arguably, the community could have withdrawn itself from those members who became 'contaminated', for it is sometimes forgotten, when discussing the fears of infection by the virus of a putative 'general population' (see, for example, Sontag 1988), that there are a large number of gay men, as well as heterosexuals, who do not have HIV. Instead, however, they chose (we suggest it was a choice, rather than necessity, as Padgug and Oppenheimer argue) first, to accept and help those affected by the illness in the early years of the epidemic (the development of services was initiated and led by a self-help movement arising from within the gay community (Weeks, 1989) and they continue to play a major role in service delivery), and second, to use AIDS as a new platform through which to promote gay liberation and gay rights. Padgug and Oppenheimer (1992) describe the process in this way:

> By owning it the (gay) community could reconstruct both the disease and its relationship to it on its own terms . . . AIDS provided a powerful and renewed source of strength to gay identity and gay institutions . . . and it created a sense of crisis that moved even the most non-political homosexuals and those whose participation in the community had hitherto been marginal to provide their money, labor and talent for the struggle.

It is of particular interest that what we see in the response of the gay community to HIV/AIDS is the extending of one ideology to encompass other ideological perspectives, notably those surrounding various aspects of caregiving. As Brown (1989) points out, ideologically based social movements, such as those promoting 'alternative' therapies, hospices, community care, self-help initiatives, or consumerism, all play major roles in the health care system. Thus, just as the middle years of this century saw a distinctively gay ideology growing out of wider social movements supporting individual liberties, civil rights and equal opportunities, so the need to develop structures and policies for a completely new and unexpected facet of gay life – mortal illness – required the adoption of ideologies current during the same period among those concerned with disabilities, chronic disease and terminal care.

The alliances formed with other social movements through the adoption of these ideologies also strengthened the position of the gay community in a number of ways. It gave access to 'experts' other than doctors, which allowed gays with HIV to challenge the traditional medical model of patient care. It also gave access to a whole new voluntary sector health care labour market, populated to a great extent by middle-class, middle-aged women (Patton 1990), without which it is difficult to see how the gay community on its own could have sustained its self-help initiatives.

Finally, and possibly most importantly of all, the new health care ideo-logies came out of what McCarthy and Wolfson (1992) characterize as a consensus rather than a conflict social movement tradition. Consensus ideologies focus on change issues that, at least in their undifferentiated form, are supported, rather than opposed, by the general population; few would, for instance, disagree with the concept of community care, whereas the concept of gay rights is less likely to be acceptable to the majority. It may be argued that the gay movement's association with the new health care ideologies made its concerns more assimilable within formal public sector bureaucracies, where, as we shall see in Chapter 6, they supplied much of the drive and energy required to develop new forms of patient care delivery.

Conservative sources of resistance

While radical social movements were providing a mobilizing source of energy towards service development in one direction, opposing these were potential sources of resistance to the new notions of personal conduct associated with liberation ideology. One should not forget how fundamen-tal a change the new type of lifestyle and the beliefs and values underpinning it represented when compared to traditionally espoused norms of Christian family life, and how shocking certain social groupings found the rapid pace of change apparent since the late 1960s. It can be argued that the advent of the Conservative government in 1979 was the outward and visible sign of an antiliberal backlash that had, until then, been relatively weak and marginalized.

'The moral majority'

Early sources of resistance to the permissive society might be traced back to origins in the fundamentalist churches and associated moral reform groups of the late Victorian era, with their notion of monogamous mar-riage as a morally privileged lifestyle and profound disapproval of hedonistic pursuits such as drug use and sexual licence. Such ideas had clearly lin-gered longer in some areas than others, and were apparently embedded in the political cultures in particular localities, such as in Scotland, where early initiatives to set up harm minimization schemes in the field of drugs services ran into opposition, which were seen by some as having its roots in Calvinism. Associated with these groupings might be 'profamily' pres-sure groups and traditionalist politicians.

The politics of moral outrage are of course not new. Wallis' (1976) analysis of the career of Mrs Mary Whitehouse as a moral entrepreneur within the vehicle of the National Viewers' and Listeners' Association in the 1960s and 1970s suggests that curbing the growth of sexual permis-siveness was – along with curbing the BBC – a major objective for the organization. The Association was construed by Wallis as a movement of cultural fundamentalism, which sought to reassert traditional values in the face of massive cultural change. Its support was seen as lying in some 'respectable' but apparently declining sectors of society (fitting Touraine's (1981) theory of social movements), which may well have gone on to form the bed-rock support of Thatcherism.

The philosophy of neoconservatism

While the 'moral majority' may, in some senses at least, have been always with us, the 1980s are often seen as characterized by the rise of the New Right as a coherent ideology, challenging the conventional social democrat wisdom of the postwar age. Most often associated with neoliberalism in the field of economic policy, a neoconservative reassessment was also evident in social policy with its notions of the underclass and dependency culture challenging the universalist prescriptions of the 1960s.

Critics such as David (1984) also saw the New Right as developing a new morality in the field of the family, with the recasting of women into traditional roles as wives and mothers, and the transfer of issues from the public to the private spheres. Such a process was being orchestrated by New Right theoreticians, centred on, for example, Peterhouse College, Cambridge and *The Salisbury Review*. In the field of sexual behaviour, Scruton (1986), as a neoconservative moral philosopher, rejects the idea that sexual behaviour should be seen solely as a social construct, rather it has a universal and moral significance, with some expressions of sexuality being praiseworthy – those that follow moral lines – while others are morally condemnable or even 'perverted'.

Although Scruton does not give a simple answer to whether homosexuality can be properly described as a perversion, it is inescapable that many applauding the rediscovery of morality in relation to sex would not be so equivocal. Mrs Thatcher's personal intervention to prevent government sponsorship of a national survey on sexual behaviour, said to have derived from 'an instinctive distaste for an invasion of heterosexual privacy' (Street 1993), can be seen as a visible manifestation of traditionalist values subscribed to, though frequently more covertly, by many older, middle-class people. There were many who felt very strongly that gay men had 'brought AIDS on themselves', and some doctors, who as a group were by no means immune from such attitudes, were sometimes reluctant to give treatment or were perceived as delivering a stigmatizing service.

Thus New Right ideology may perhaps be seen as adding an intellectual gloss, and therefore greater respectability to the traditionalist moral attitudes espoused by such as Mary Whitehouse, and the large Conservative majorities in the 1983 and 1987 Parliaments might at first glance be thought to represent favourable terrain for these forces. Indeed the passing into law of Section 28, which made it an offence for local government to 'promote homosexuality', supports this argument. However, the influence of conservative sources of resistance on the response to the HIV/AIDS epidemic seems to have been weakened by the liberal forces described earlier: they were the dogs that did not bark. Testing represented a symbolic issue, yet calls for compulsory testing were always rejected by government.

The relevance of ideology to the development of HIV/AIDS services

We saw in Chapter 3 that the characteristics of the key settings in which HIV/AIDS services developed, both affected and were themselves affected, by the issue. We argue here that, in the same way, the various ideological stances espoused by different groups in society both influenced the response and were, sometimes very fundamentally, modified by it.

Ideologies have both an *interpretive* function, offering a framework through which an issue can be understood, and also a link with *action* (either movement or immobility). Where their interpretive function is concerned, it is important to note here that the four identifiable general ideological perspectives we described in the last section are not necessarily mutually exclusive in relation to individuals. Hence a doctor, while looking at HIV/AIDS from the standpoint of a professional approach to dealing with disease, could also take a conservative and moralistic attitude towards the patient, or, alternatively, be in sympathy with the ideals of gay liberation.

Linking ideologies with action brings in the concept of 'mind sets', as the application of ideologies to particular aspects of the environment, rather than just as general ways of thinking about the world. So we look at some of the effects of ideologically constructed mind sets on how people responded to the need for action posed by HIV/AIDS. We also consider how ideologies can trigger a release of energy, sustaining an issue even in the face of opposition.

The interpretive role of ideologies

Ideologies and attitudes to disease

'AIDS' says Berridge (1993) 'now has its own history, rather than borrowing from the more distant past'; but for some time the past was the only way in which this totally new issue could be understood, and how the past was seen depended on many different perspectives. For instance, the terms 'epidemic' and 'infection' could mean various things depending on one's viewpoint. For hospital personnel dealing with patients, HIV/AIDS was seen as a control of cross-infection issue, with staff dressed in 'spacesuits' evoking, at one and the same time, the plagues of the middle ages (Sontag 1988) and present-day concerns about radioactive fall-out. For professionals like public health physicians, on the other hand, epidemics were a key part of their professional expertise, not so much something frightening as something exciting and stimulating – a new challenge they were equipped to meet. The comment of one of our respondents that 'It would have been a pity not to be part of the only proper epidemic this century' typifies this attitude.

For government ministers the advent of HIV/AIDS suggested the need for the imposition of controls, and they hurried to update the Public Health (Infectious Diseases) Regulations to allow the detention of people with AIDS if they could be identified as putting others at risk. However, the only time this was implemented (in Manchester in March 1985) such a furore ensued from those whose values stressed the importance of civil liberties that the Act has never been invoked since.

Ideologies and moral attitudes

The whole history surrounding sexually transmitted diseases has moral overtones, with a tendency to apportion 'blame' in the transmission of infection (generally to women rather than men), and some groups making repeated attempts to regulate forms of sexual deviance such as promiscuity, prostitution and homosexuality. This contrasted with the attitude taken by some, not just during the so-called 'permissive' 1960s but between the wars, celebrating freedom in sexual relationships and trivializing associated infections.

Drug use, as we discussed in Chapter 3, had similarly been the subject of ideological 'swings and roundabouts' over a long period. Drug dependency is clinically defined as a branch of psychiatry. Reflecting the more general growth of sociological critiques of medicine in the 1960s, this label has been fiercely contested by 'antipsychiatrists' such as Szasz (1975), who feel that the case for psychiatric intervention has not been made and that rather drug dependence is a social problem that has been subject to unwarranted medicalization.

The historical process by which the drugs 'problem' underwent a process of medicalization has been outlined by Berridge and Edwards (1981) as the Victorian concept of the use of drugs such as opiates as a 'bad habit' was gradually replaced by a concept of 'addiction'. As they also argue, another profoundly important development was the criminalization of drug use after the 1920 Dangerous Drug Use Act made the possession of opiates a criminal offence and brought in the Home Office, setting up a debate between illness-based and control-based views of policy. This also brought the beginnings of an alliance between medical 'experts' and the bureaucracy of control, which goes forward to the Home Office's Advisory Council on the Misuse of Drugs (Berridge and Edwards 1981: 253).

It has been suggested by some that religious bigotry may have been responsible for some of the intransigent attitudes towards gay people and drug use that characterized the early years of the epidemic, but in fact the evidence, which indicates that church-based organizations were early in the field, suggests the opposite. A plausible interpretation of the paradox was posited by one of our respondents, a public health physician:

> There is a moral climate in any country which is not just religious but it's moral, it's non-religious, it's ethical, it's legal . . . the whole basis for a culture is more than just religion. I'm sure that religion plays a part but it's attitudes that were formed three or four hundred years ago, so it's not as simple as what the church does now.

Ideologies and knowledge

As the comment on the development of the response to drug use makes clear, what was seen as 'knowledge' in the field of HIV/AIDS was also affected by ideological perspectives. Boudon (1989: 143) points out that 'scientific knowledge is not only not protected from beliefs which are not proven, it could not even exist without them'. The particular value system of medical science has a long history and, despite its popular image as dealing in 'facts', represents an ideology based around a belief in the supremacy of a hypotheticodeductive approach and in a biomedical model, which ignores social contextual factors (Mishler 1981). However, at a normative level a range of sharply conflicting value systems is apparent. There have even been profound epistemological questions raised in debate, such as whether scientific knowledge has a privileged status in relation to experiential knowledge. Theorists coming out of social movements indeed emphasize the primacy of the lived experience as a source of knowledge. Patton (1990: Chapter 3) takes up this point:

> Simultaneous with the emergence of institutions to deliver AIDS services was the formation of a set of 'AIDS knowledges', . . . the 'experts' knew about the virus and treatment, the 'person living with AIDS' knew about suffering and death, the 'volunteer' knew about the courage of the human spirit.

Ideologies and policies

Particular specialties within professional groupings also demonstrated ideological mind sets enshrined as policy. For instance, patient confidentiality has always been an important feature of genitourinary medicine services for obvious reasons of patient stigma, and has remained a strong part of the culture of the specialty. With HIV/AIDS there is a persistent tension between an individual patient's desire for confidentiality and the needs of others:

> Confidentiality is a real problem, there is a real trade-off between confidentiality and effective prevention . . . [but] . . . if you said, 'nobody can be assured of any confidentiality, we will pursue you with

all the resources available, you are going to get visited at home, your GP is going to be told, everybody is going to know, your sexual partners are going to know—'. That's fine, but the immediate effect would be to drive it underground, people wouldn't want to come forward.

(public health physician respondent)

In health promotion, also, the approach to HIV/AIDS tended to be mediated by a particular ideological stance. The three traditional models of health education – behaviour change, self-empowerment and collective action (French and Adams 1986) – have been, suggest Homans and Aggleton (1988) supplanted in the case of HIV/AIDS by a *social transformatory* model combining elements of each. The model was heavily influenced by its inheritance from the voluntary sector, where SMOs such as the Terrence Higgins Trust had established a track-record of health promotion work. Its further development can be seen as producing a far-reaching agenda for social change, which went far beyond the usual remit of health promotion initiatives.

Lack of policies could also be seen as resulting from an ideological perspective. Hence a strong belief in the conquest of infectious disease had so permeated the medical community that ordinary safeguards had come to be ignored. Even after the advent of HIV/AIDS such mind sets sometimes proved extremely difficult to change, as newly appointed control of cross-infection staff discovered when they tried to convince nurses and doctors to take precautions with blood and body fluids.

The role of ideologies in mediating action

Ideologies and decision-making

Organizational decision-making in this field above all – we argue – was shaped not only by formal structure, flows of resources or the more anaemic conception of organizational 'culture', but by the formation of, and contest between, quite different ideologies of personal conduct, sometimes articulated at the level of formal theory, but also apparent in a broader 'theory in use' among particular constituencies.

We thus see a number of very different value systems in coexistence and in conflict. At a national level, perhaps unexpectedly, we argue that at least within the process of decision-making within the NHS, the interpretation advanced by a liberal/radical alliance between some individual clinicians, much of public health and the gay social movement generally proved dominant over the ideas advanced by the more conservative grouping of a putative 'moral majority' and New Right theoreticians.

However, if the liberals by and large succeeded in imposing their view of appropriate policy on government, this did not always immediately translate to practice at organizational level. There were certainly examples of the potential of HIV/AIDS to mediate existing policy: the setting up of needle exchanges and adoption of a harm minimization policy for drug users, new doctor–patient relationships and changes in infection control measures. One interesting example of just how powerful the perceived imperatives could be came from a respondent in a social services department who found himself forced to reconsider long-standing ideologies about appropriate childcare: 'I had to have a contingency plan drawn up to re-open shut-down children's homes and to re-invent the residential nursery, a thing that all my generation spent time stamping out.'

Nevertheless there was also evidence of many who firmly clung to cherished policies. For instance, many long-standing staff who had grown up with the abstinence-based models of the 1970s found it difficult to adopt the new harm minimization approach to drug use now being advocated. Meanwhile, new groupings of staff, often younger, more radical and with a background in the voluntary sector, rejected medically led models and had a firm attachment to the new approach.

Symbolism and ideologies
There were certain concrete manifestations of this ideological hegemony, such as the new language system that arose to describe HIV/AIDS (see Thompson (1984) for a discussion of the study of the role of language within ideology). People's value systems and extent to which they were in touch with those working in the field at grass roots level could often be inferred from their choice of words: should one refer to 'drug addicts', 'drug misusers' or 'drug injectors' for instance? As for the term 'junkies', that could only be used at a jocular level, which made it perfectly clear that you understood that the term was inappropriate. The pervasive and compelling nature of the new linguistic norms, which emerged as 'outward and visible' signs of what those who perpetrated them hoped were new 'inward and spiritual' values, was finally acknowledged by the Health Education Authority, which issued a list of 'acceptable' HIV/AIDS vocabulary: 'person with AIDS', for example, was to be preferred to 'AIDS sufferer'.

New topic areas were opened up for acceptable discussion. Often the office walls of HIV/AIDS staff would be covered with well-designed and frequently very explicit visual material (such as posters celebrating safe sex). This, with the plentiful supplies of leaflets and condoms, reinforced a certain set of images. 'Condom talk' has become far more acceptable socially in the late 1980s, reflecting perhaps some of these processes.

As we have seen, HIV/AIDS was associated, particularly initially, with strong feelings of fear and stigma and overtones of moral depravity. Did a hospital want to become known as an 'AIDS centre'? Turning the image of the issue round was an important task for some actors, and was achieved with some success in a number of the localities. Association with high status 'patrons' was also important. The photograph of the Princess of Wales opening the new AIDS ward at the Middlesex Hospital, for example, and shaking hands with the patients, went round the world and did much to change the image of the issue there. The royal laying on of hands is, of course, an act historically charged with special meaning, with 'good' triumphing over 'evil'.

Achieving commitment

How to secure and maintain energy and commitment over a very long time-period is a central problem in organizational change processes (such as responding to the HIV/AIDS epidemic). How did a health care issue associated with marginal social groupings come to be placed high on the formal policy agenda and the momentum maintained after the political limelight had moved on to other issues? Essentially short-term sources of energy, such as charismatic leadership, are unlikely to be enough. We know that ideological belief systems may play an extremely important role in defining a social grouping, impelling it to action through mobilization, structuring its external relations and also acting as way of controlling adherents (Pettigrew 1979). In many organizations, allegiance may be voluntary rather than as part of a wage contract or membership of a total institution, so control through a shared belief system assumes particular prominence. It is therefore unsurprising that the term 'ideology' features prominently in analyses of many different value laden organizations as a glue which holds them together.

The following account typifies many such groups in the field of HIV/AIDS:

> There existed within [the group] a definite group 'culture', and a sense of cohesion which are hard to define precisely, but which derive from a general and implicitly recognized sharing of certain political, social and cultural beliefs and attitudes. This resulted in a high level of commitment both to the work of the Group and the Group itself.
> (Kleiman 1989)

Often the possession of a strong and energizing ideology is seen as an important resource for a group. Moss Kanter (1972), in her examination of nineteenth century American communes and utopias, concluded that, for a group to survive, a corporate ideology was needed to legitimate demands made on members with reference to a higher principle. Comments made by respondents from some of the organizations that developed in response to HIV/AIDS suggest that such groups equally reflected a sense of mission – 'when I started I was evangelical'; 'I think that was my platform, that it was important that the homophobia, racism and sexism were confronted'.

Moss Kanter noted that groups that could generate and sustain high levels of commitment tended to last, and that such longevity indicated a functioning social order, whereas the unsuccessful communities often fell apart at the first crisis. Successful groups could display considerable powers of determination: 'Their devotion and will to survive weathered economic crises, physical relocations, natural disasters ranging from fires and famines to disease, societal persecution, internal dissension and even crises of leadership succession' (Moss Kanter 1972). The continuing survival of the Terrence Higgins Trust, despite experiencing most of these vicissitudes (Schramm-Evans 1990), is a testament to the strength of ideological commitment of such present-day SMOs.

Concluding remarks

In summary, we suggest in this chapter that some quite distinctive ideological perspectives are identifiable amongst some of the key social groupings exerting influence on the development of services for HIV/AIDS and we argue that recognition of what might be termed 'the ideological context of HIV/AIDS' is essential to understanding the organizational response.

Strong (1990) has already explored some aspects of the psychology of an epidemic, focusing on the destabilizing effect of great uncertainty on organizational behaviour. Certainly HIV/AIDS cannot be seen solely as a neutral or technical issue but as one that was highly charged politically, morally and intellectually, as well as emotionally.

Ideology helped to stabilize the situation and reduce the level of uncertainty to a tolerable level. Very different accounts were accessed of the nature of the epidemic, supplying very different interpretations of what had happened at a policy level, as well as suggesting alternative preferred courses of action. A struggle for interpretation was going on. Any analysis of the response to the HIV/AIDS epidemic by health care organizations must then consider subjective factors that are rather different from those addressed by the broad and relatively anaemic concept of 'organizational culture' so popular in the 1980s.

What we see in the response to HIV/AIDS is that ideologies and beliefs arose more than were shaped. The ideologies and systems of thought outlined were embedded societally and historically, rather than organizationally specific or created by top management. Some important shifts in group consciousness were outlined, which helped explain how world views changed. This in turn helped explain the ambiguous relationship between key groups in the epidemic, such as the gay social movement and professionals practising biomedicine.

Many accounts of ideology have stressed its negative features, such as intolerance, zealotry, and the danger of groupthink (Janis 1968). Exclusive groups may be too ready to label outsiders and thus make attempts to form wider coalitions more difficult, and energy may be used in promoting a narrow range of sacred policies. Groups may become fixated on particular ways of addressing issues, despite evidence that they were not effective and dismissive of alternative approaches. HIV/AIDS was a complex and difficult problem, compounded by the difficulty that to start with 'no one knew anything' (Strong and Berridge 1990). These are exactly the conditions under which people rely more than ever on ways in which they have previously construed the world to decide their courses of action, necessitating, as Turner (1976) in his analysis of the development of disasters points out, 'the collective adoption of simplifying assumptions about the environment' that: '. . . offer a way of deciding what to ignore in a more complex formulation to produce a statement of the problem in which uncertainty has been reduced.'

While these are real dangers, this chapter has also examined the positive and affirming role that a group ideology can play in raising energy levels around change, raising issues on agendas, acquiring political support and ensuring long-range commitment. Such strong belief systems may substitute for structure as a form of organizational glue. These belief systems were, however, most apparent in gay SMOs, where flows of financial and political support seemed stronger than (say) in the drugs field.

Clearly the construction of language systems, metaphors and tropes are an important part of the creation of the AIDS discourse. Sontag (1988) has analysed and criticized the notion of 'plague' as the principal metaphor through which AIDS was understood in its early days. A whole new language system and forms of visual imagery indeed arose to describe HIV/AIDS. But alongside this focus on meaning, ideology also acted to purvey doctrine, for example, the borrowing by gay liberation theory of concepts from the New Left or from feminism.

Are there general conclusions to be drawn from all this? First, we hope to have convinced the reader of the important role played by ideologies in mediating behaviour at individual, group and organizational level, and that any analysis of organizational change ignores ideological issues at the expense of omitting a key influence on situations.

Second, we would argue strongly for a perspective that recognizes ideologies as part of the external, as well as the internal context of organizations and that historical, as well as contemporary contexts should be taken into account.

The third and final point relates to the source of ideologies. Although many analyses see ideology within organizations as being imposed from above, often through a key change agent such as a new chief executive, our data suggest that ideology may just as frequently be a 'bottom-up' phenomenon, triggered by wider social movements and introduced through small groups and coalitions of like-minded people.

Given the lack of recognized cause/effect relationships, the scale of the HIV/AIDS issue, and its profound social and indeed moral implications, it is unsurprising that ideological belief systems often stepped into an apparent vacuum, offering individuals at least some guide to action. Much social and political conflict centres on change, and here the existence of coherent belief systems may be important in guiding action thought to lead to a desired state of affairs (Seliger, 1976). As Pettigrew (1979) puts it:

New organizations thus represent settings where it is possible to study transition processes from no beliefs to new beliefs, from no rules to new rules, from no culture to new culture and in general terms to observe the translation of ideas into structural and expressive forms.

We suggest that the new organizations created by the response to HIV/ AIDS can represent a fruitful area for investigation of the construction and role of organizational ideologies.

CHAPTER
5

Issue recognition – the stimulus for innovation

Introduction

We have seen in Chapter 4 that the response to HIV/AIDS was influenced by the presence of a variety of alternative and indeed competing ideologies. In this chapter we start to look in detail at some of the change processes studied, particularly understanding how a new issue gains attention and becomes important within an organization.

Much of the organizational literature on innovation has concentrated on processes whereby a new idea takes hold either because it offers a solution to a previously expressed problem or, as described in Cohen et al.'s (1972) 'garbage can' model of organizational choice, because the idea is so clearly a solution that it is worthwhile identifying an issue it can address. March (1988) suggests that these models of the innovation process are very different, the one being stimulated by the need to take rational and purposive action to deal with perceived need, and the other resulting from there being sufficient leeway or 'slack' within the organization for new ideas to generate. However, what these models have in common is that both address the underlying need of the organization or parts of the organization to improve performance within already identified strategic objectives.

The second type of innovation process, less frequently addressed in the management literature until recently, results from a perception of a need to change or extend organizational objectives to address qualitatively different and unexpected environmental stimuli. Here, as exemplified by the

HIV/AIDS issue, the driving force for innovation and change comes from outside. This means that the organization has first to recognize or 'sense' (Lyles 1981) the existence of the issue, which may be difficult without previous experience of anything similar, and second, the organization must accept the need for innovation.

Here, we are essentially analysing the very first stages of a long-term change process in which new and possibly threatening information is acquired by organizational actors; this information then leads them to embark upon social and organizational action. Strong (1990) offers one account of the peculiar social psychology of the early stages of an epidemic, suggesting that there may be rapid mood shifts as waves of anxiety and panic go round the organization. On the other hand, this opens the way to those who have clear 'solutions' to offer as there is an increasing clamour for action.

Other accounts operate from a more explicit focus on how actors within organizations sense new problems. For instance, Johnston's (1975) model of the organizational change process usefully distinguishes between four stages:

1 the development of concern;
2 the acknowledgement and understanding of the problem;
3 planning and acting;
4 stabilizing change.

On the basis of his analysis of the process of strategic change in ICI, Pettigrew (1985: 473) has noted the role of visionary leaders and early adopters in change processes, indicating the importance of an initial problem-sensing stage, which may predate the development of widespread concern throughout the organization. In the sphere of change, even signalling problems as worthy of attention and getting those problems discussed is a time-consuming and politically sensitive process. Such pioneers may either be individuals or indeed small groups operating with more of a team approach.

So, in looking at how groups and organizations recognized and responded to HIV/AIDS we are also addressing an issue with more general application within organization studies, namely: how are new, unusual and difficult problems sensed by organizational actors? In this chapter, we consider the response of existing formal organizations (the NHS, social services departments) rather than single issue based voluntary organizations for whom perceiving the importance of the new issue was much less problematic.

The organizational and political context in which the HIV/AIDS issue arose

We here discuss briefly two aspects of the context; both exerted important negative influences on the issue recognition process.

The density of the management agenda and the financial situation

The process of raising awareness of HIV/AIDS can be seen as being modified not only by the nature of the issue itself, but also by the context in which it arose. Thus an important historical influence on service development within the NHS was the density of the managerial agenda in each health authority, which was intimately associated with the local financial situation.

Although there was some local variation, the broad scenario was much the same in all our authorities – a picture of increasing financial stringency since the mid-1970s and increasing managerial control dating from the implementation of general management following the Griffiths Report in 1983 (DHSS 1983b). This led in particular to problems of financial control in stressed acute sector budgets, which soaked up much senior managerial time. In one authority, at least one early application for research that might have thrown some light on immune deficiency in haemophiliacs was turned down. In another, although the existence of HIV had been recognized, those who wanted to determine the size of the local problem had their efforts frustrated for six months by the health authority's unwillingness to allocate money to set up a testing service:

> There were resources needed for setting up a service for HIV testing. There was a lot of reluctance to parting with the money [between the various possible funding bodies] ... each wanted the other to pay ... There was a general reluctance to provide money ... and as I say, a lot of time and effort was expended by people to try and get things going. In retrospect they were fairly trivial sums of money, £10,000 or £20,000.
>
> (health service respondent)

Under these financial circumstances, it was difficult to raise money for anything new within the health authorities. As we shall see later, individuals and groups in authorities that responded early found ways of circumventing these difficulties, but in the years before the government made special funding available the financial climate in the NHS undoubtedly inhibited progress in responding to HIV/AIDS.

Local variation in the organization of the public health function and health/local authority collaboration

The reorganizations of health and local government during the 1970s and early 1980s had affected some of our authorities more than others. In some, boundaries had remained unchanged, facilitating continuity of relationships. In others, area health authorities that had been coterminous with local authorities were split into districts sharing an urban area with a number of other authorities. This made liaison and cooperation, both with other health authorities, and with the local authority and voluntary groups, much more complex.

As noted earlier, one of the disciplines most affected by these changes was public health, where roles had become increasingly confused since the function had been split between health and local authorities at the inception of the NHS. The 1982 reorganization left some of the new district health authorities (DHAs) without a functioning department concerned with public health, just at a time when there was a clear need for a strong public health lead in raising awareness of the wider relevance of the HIV/AIDS issue.

In one of our authorities, the public health physician, though he was later to become a key figure in the field and the motivating influence on the development of HIV/AIDS services, had been so involved in building a public health department from scratch that it was not until he attended a conference in 1985 that he really became aware of the need to address the issue:

> I remember sitting there . . . thinking . . . 'It's really down to me to go and do something about it.' . . . So I thought 'Well OK, if I am going to do something, what is it I do?' and I didn't know. So I thought 'well, I'd better inform myself' . . . So for about three or four months at the beginning of 1985 I read a lot and went to a lot of conferences about HIV, and by the summer I felt I wasn't learning anything new; I knew as much as I could find out at that stage and I had the general shape of things in my mind, and thought 'Well, I'd better do something about it'.

This situation affected all our case study authorities to a greater or lesser degree, and probably explains the relatively low profile of public health physicians in the very early years of the epidemic.

In a few of our authorities, public health was heavily involved in raising awareness of the HIV/AIDS issue from the very beginning. In one, conditions were particularly favourable. Reorganization had not affected health authority boundaries; there was a strong tradition of public health going right back to the nineteenth century, which had to a great extent survived in spite of the mutating roles imposed upon those employed in the discipline; and there was a history of cooperation with the local authority over health issues. Finally, and probably most importantly of all, a key appointment of a consultant in public health who was also an epidemiologist, was fortuitously made in early 1983, providing someone who was both available and able to take a lead role on the issue. All this gave the authority a head start in recognizing and responding to the HIV/AIDS issue, despite having very few early cases of AIDS. This was one of the few examples amongst our case study authorities of the HIV/AIDS issue being recognized and taken up as a controlled and strategically organized managerial and organizational process from a very early stage.

Becoming aware of HIV/AIDS

Having seen the effect of some general contextual factors on the development of awareness of HIV/AIDS as a new and important health care issue, we now move on to consider some of the other factors, many of them inherent in the nature of HIV/AIDS itself, which led to early recognition of the issue in our authorities.

To some extent the recognition of HIV/AIDS as an issue was a temporal process affecting not only healthcare workers and health authorities but other organizations, the government and the general public. This was a genuinely new situation and there was a progression over time from the awareness of a few to the awareness of the many, and also from HIV/AIDS being seen as something of concern to only very specific aspects of an organization or a community, to the acknowledgement that HIV/AIDS was of general importance. First – at least within NHS settings – came the very early sensing of a new issue of scientific interest, involving only a very few specialist researchers and having few immediate consequences for patients or for the organization as a whole. Then came the beginnings of awareness of the relevance of HIV/AIDS to particular groups of patients and specific specialties, and to the staff who had to deal with them. Finally, as a sense of crisis and urgency began to build, came awareness that HIV/AIDS was going to be an issue that affected not only every aspect of health care organizations, but many other organizations as well, and that it had profound implications for the future health of the population as a whole.

This temporal progression in the process of issue recognition was affected, in our early responding health authorities, by a number of other contextual factors, some which speeded the process and others which tended to inhibit. Some of these are listed below:

- Sensing the issue:
  - a 'scientific' organizational culture;
  - existing service provision in key specialties;
  - emerging social movement organizations.
- Raising awareness within the organization:
  - individuals' perceptions of potential local prevalence;
  - confirmed cases of HIV and AIDS;
  - staff anxieties;
  - creation of specialist resources.
- Recognizing the importance and wider relevance of the issue:
  - the local social and political climate.

In the next three sections we consider these factors and the roles they played in the development of awareness of HIV/AIDS and initiating action in the health authorities we studied.

Sensing the issue

A 'scientific' organizational culture

One important factor in facilitating the recognition of HIV/AIDS in our DHAs was what may be described as a 'big acute hospital culture'. Many were health authorities in large university cities and contained several major acute hospitals; they were also often teaching authorities. In such settings are traditionally found the medical specialists who are at the forefront of their professions, are involved in research programmes of their own and who take a keen interest in the latest developments in their specialties throughout the world. It was amongst this group that the first glimmerings of medical awareness of a new health problem began. One respondent, a consultant haematologist, remembered:

> I began to wonder whether there was a possibility that they were immunocompromised . . . as early as '79 . . . Through one of my other interests, leukaemia, I was at a workshop in Washington when the first cases of Kaposi's sarcoma were presented in homosexuals.

That was before the first reports of cases of AIDS were published in 1981, but others were aware of the issue almost as early: 'I was aware that it was going to be hitting Britain even in '81/'82 because I've been an avid reader of MMWR[1] . . . so as soon as HIV came on the horizon I certainly knew about it.'

Initially no-one was even certain that an infective agent was involved, and it was mainly immunologists who were interested in the syndrome, but the established traditions of medical and scientific research ensured that the early cases of AIDS were recognized as 'something new' and, for this very reason, worthy of study. Something was in the air within the leading-edge research community, and key players were using their international networks to take first steps, such as setting up cohort studies to gather basic epidemiological data, as this comment from a leading London hospital in 1983 makes clear: 'I think the idea of a cohort just came out of an interaction thing . . . we were aware that the American cohorts had started, it seemed a very obvious thing to do.'

This early sensing of the issue, then, owed far more to the general mind set of the scientific elite, what Roe (1952) in her study of the personal attributes of scientists characterized as 'the need to find out', than to prescience about the future importance of AIDS. Sometimes, as in this case, such curiosity-driven research goes on to have an unexpected degree of direct policy relevance.

In 1983 it became clear that the breakdown of the immune system that characterized AIDS was caused by a sexually transmissible virus, now known as human immunodeficiency virus (HIV). There is still bitter argument and a legal wrangle over whether an American or French scientist actually made this discovery (Connor 1992) but now a different grouping, the virologists, became involved in the issue. As Shilts (1987) argues, we should remember that interest in the HIV/AIDS issue was being generated at least as much by competition amongst scientists for the kudos involved in being credited with a new discovery, as by 'pure' scientific curiosity. Leading-edge scientists and directors of research units need to be seen in part as 'academic entrepreneurs' as well as disinterested seekers after truth.

Certainly, following identification of the HIV virus, all over the world the race was on to develop a diagnostic test. One leading virology department studied knew that it was in competition with other research groups in developing a marker test and that it had to move quickly. Early approaches to the MRC for funds were unsuccessful, with the result that the virologists themselves were undertaking the bulk of the work during the summer of 1984 'out of hours', and with little back-up from specially funded staff, who only arrived later. There were, however, organizational costs associated with this breakneck pace of research and a crisis blew up within the department over disregard of safety procedures; this came close to destroying the department.

This quotation from a virologist in another hospital we studied captures the excitement of the scientific chase generated at this time:

> From the very first finding of the HIV virus, I think we were probably the first laboratory in this country to be able to diagnose the disease. We got a copy of the subculture from Porton, and we started doing tests ourselves of a very simple nature which we devised . . . from the very earliest days, so much so I broke all the rules in the book by using Gallo's [one of the virologists involved in the initial isolation of HIV] strain, even though at that stage he was claiming to have it patented and people weren't allowed to use it. So I used it and said 'Sue me if you will'.

The doctor quoted in this example had little direct involvement with patients. For others, however, there was less of a distinction between research and clinical concerns. Another aspect of the medical scientific culture in our authorities that tended to facilitate early awareness of the issue was that the application of expertise in one area sometimes led to early recognition of a problem in another.

Thus in 1982 one consultant sought and obtained research funding to investigate the possibility of immune suppression in haemophiliacs, after noticing that his patients with haemophilia were much more susceptible to tuberculosis than others. When the first diagnostic tests for HIV were being developed he had sequential serum samples already available, allowing early identification of HIV infection among his patients. Similarly, testing the samples of blood serum stored by doctors with a scientific research interest in the spread of hepatitis B amongst drug users (Peutherer et al. 1985; Robertson et al. 1986) led to the early realization that some localities had a very large incidence of HIV infection amongst this group of patients.

Many of the authorities studied were financially advantaged in comparison with other authorities in their regions, and had been so for many years. This skewed distribution of resources reflected both recognition of a net inflow of patients from other authorities and also the traditional support given to 'high tech' medicine (Hunter 1980; Strong and Robinson 1990). It was expected and legitimate for doctors to pursue their own research interests. To some extent, therefore, even in the conditions of increasing financial stringency of the early 1980s, there was space within the system for investigating new issues, the organizational slack, which, as noted earlier, Cohen and March (1974) identified as an important facilitator for innovation.

However, the relative status and autonomy of some of the interested medical consultants enabled them to use their discretion to vire resources to pump-prime projects:

> The way I view what happened is that part of it is interest and part of it is having enough resources at your disposal that you can channel through and switch and say, 'right we're going to go for this because its important' . . . And once the demand set in it was very difficult for [the health authority] to say, 'hang on, you can't do this', which is what they would have done if I hadn't gone to [X] and said I'd like an afternoon clinic.
>
> (clinical product champion)

Thus, early development of services did not necessarily result from recognition of the HIV problem at an organizational level. It was in part due to individuals having what Pfeffer and Salancik (1978) characterized as resource power, the ability to control the discretionary use of funds to further something they thought was important.

So the very early sensing of the HIV/AIDS issue within the NHS came about primarily as a result of individual interest and, in some cases, personal ambition; but was assisted by organizational factors such as relatively more favourable resourcing and a culture in which entrepreneurial activity was legitimate.

Pre-existing specialties – an infrastructure for service development

Although some of those early in sensing the new issue worked almost exclusively within laboratory medicine, most carried a clinical workload as well as being involved in research. Although it was not immediately clear how, or even if, AIDS resulted from infection by a virus, early clues from the first patients affected pointed to probable links with either sexual activity, and/or contaminated blood products. It was therefore mainly within the clinical medical specialties of genitourinary medicine, haemophilia and infectious diseases that clinicians were first reading about and becoming interested in the new disease.

Early sensing of an issue is of course unlikely to occur in a vacuum. In all our authorities, the early recognition of the HIV/AIDS issue came from within some kind of appropriate service infrastructure, which served as an essential focus for issue recognition and early service development. Early patients with AIDS were admitted to these wards, or identified in these clinics, enabling cohort studies to be set up. Once tests for the virus were available these departments were frequently seen as the obvious places to base testing clinics and the associated counselling services.

However, the role played by existing services in facilitating issue recognition was not purely that of providing the means whereby interested clinicians could pursue their research. As we have already noted, prior to HIV/AIDS none of the key specialties was a major contender for prestige and influence within the health authorities. Some of those who took action early were prompted as much, or even more, by the recognition that here was something that could be used to put their specialty on the map, as by scientific interest and curiosity in the syndrome itself.

In one health authority, the facilities provided by the department of genitourinary medicine had been under severe and constant criticism for twenty years. Plans for a new department had been documented in the regional strategy since 1979, and in the capital programme since 1984, but it was not until HIV/AIDS focused attention on the specialty that work started on actually building the new premises and moves were commenced to establish a professorial chair in genitourinary medicine.

The same sort of thing was happening in other places:

> We needed to expand the sort of facilities that we had . . . they were very basic, they were very cramped, they were very unwelcoming . . . so we had plans . . . going way back, and really AIDS caught us . . . our view was the demand for the STD services was going to increase and therefore we had to be better set up in terms of space . . . We virtually doubled the size of the department.

Infectious diseases was another specialty for which HIV provided a shot in the arm. One respondent recalled: 'That [infectious diseases] unit was under considerable threat of disappearing, the whole hospital was, pre-HIV.'

Instead, early recognition that they needed to prepare for an influx of HIV-infected patients led to expansion, rather than contraction of the unit.

What we see here, then, is a coming together of two important motivating factors for change. First the exercising of research interest within
a scientific culture that both emphasized the importance and relevance of
new knowledge for its own sake, and also as part of the politics of advancement. In addition, the coincidence that HIV/AIDS was relevant to,
and offered an opportunity for expanding, specific specialties whose protagonists had long sought to establish better standing within the medical
hierarchy.

The emergence of social movement organizations
Up to this point, our analysis has concentrated on elements in the 'official'
medical/academic system that were early in the field in sensing that a new
and unusual problem was about to break. We argue that such forces were
at work from very early on in the lifecycle of the epidemic, trying to define
the emergent problem.

Writers such as Patton (1990) grossly underestimate the role played by
doctors and scientists in taking early action, albeit in the context of their
medicalized discourse. However, Patton is correct in arguing that grass-
roots (often gay) organizations were also mobilizing to place the HIV/
AIDS issue on the public agenda from the early 1980s onwards, at first in
the absence of government funding. These were groupings that sprang up
more or less spontaneously, reflecting rising levels of concern amongst the
communities most affected by the epidemic. In their early phase, they were
creative, fluid and even chaotic organizations with few formal management
systems. The Terrence Higgins Trust is a good example of the type of national SMO that sprang up in the early 1980s. Its history is presented by
Schramm-Evans (1990: 222) and is discussed in more depth in Chapter 4.

Despite apparently profound internal contradictions, the organization
enjoyed a high media profile, well-recognized spokespersons and apparent
influence on policy making at a national level (Strong and Berridge 1990).
The Terrence Higgins Trust perhaps also acted as a template for a range
of regionally based voluntary organizations, which sprang up from the
mid-1980s onwards. Our own view is that such SMOs generally appear to
have had more impact in raising awareness of HIV/AIDS at Department
of Health level and at ward or clinic level than in the middle of the NHS
hierarchy. However, as we shall see in the next section, in some of our cases,
members of such organizations had links with health authorities and played
an important role in sensitizing those in influential positions to the issue.

Awareness of the local situation

Individuals' perceptions of local risk from HIV/AIDS
As the previous section makes clear, actors drawn into the field in the early
1980s had a variety of motivations. Some sprang from the communities

most affected, or possibly had the virus themselves. Others of those early in sensing the issue had a strong interest in unravelling the scientific puzzle, and/or in enhancing the prestige of their particular specialties. However, there were also those for whom a key trigger factor was, or was also, an awareness, long before any actual patients appeared on the scene, of the need to try to reduce the risk posed by HIV/AIDS to their local population. These early movers were all very much in the minority, for, as these comments indicate, denial of the importance of the issue was widespread in the early days of the epidemic:

> I can remember very much a feeling . . . this isn't relevant to us, this isn't relevant to our work and it's unlikely to be relevant to anything that we'll do in the future. And I think that that was a feeling that pervaded for quite some considerable time.
>
> (health service respondent)

> I think there was very much an attitude of 'its not happening'. Yes, and if it was they didn't want anything to do with it. It was very much like that.
>
> (health service respondent)

Even public health physicians, who might have been expected to take the prospect of an epidemic very seriously, were not all early in accepting the need to take action. However, in support of Meyers' (1986) assertion that most crises provide opportunities, a degree of organizational disarray in public health allowed some public health physicians room to develop in new directions. HIV/AIDS represented the first major health issue for many years for which public health clearly had some responsibility, and in a number of our cases a particular public health physician ended up taking a key managerial role. None the less, though some in this specialty reacted early, others, exposed to the same information, did not, as this respondent, a public health physician, recalled:

> Certainly by mid-1983 we were debating it, saying was it going to be significant or not. And I have to say . . . [my colleague] was saying 'We've got to do something, we've got to do something, it is going to be very significant', and I was saying 'Are you sure?' And I have to say I was wrong and he was right.

Then there were often idiosyncratic reasons why some people became convinced of the urgency of the situation. A district health promotion officer, for instance, became alerted to some of the issues involved in HIV/ AIDS through her previous work in sexual counselling. A gay genitourinary medicine physician had a keen personal as well as professional concern about the risks involved in some homosexual activities. In two separate cases secretaries in public health departments became so interested in the issue that, before leaving to take up posts with local voluntary organizations concerned with HIV/AIDS, they had had a major influence on their departments. One ran an AIDS information resource library, the other used her position to expedite the progress of documents relating to the issue, as her manager recalled: '[My secretary] also got taken up by this . . . which kept it on the agenda in this department, if you like, and ensured that if things came in they did reach me urgently.'

One general practitioner with a long-standing interest in the clinical problems of drug users found himself a *de facto* authority on the subject when a large number of his patients were found to be infected. In another case, the personal experience of the head of a small hospital department made him determine to do all he could to raise the profile of the issue within his health authority:

> I brought it to [the Director of Public Health's] attention that it [AIDS] was here in [the city] . . . a friend of mine died under mysterious circumstances, eventually it was diagnosed as pneumocystis . . . he was one of the first people in [the city] but it didn't go down in the statistics because he died of pneumonia . . . so I approached [the Director of Public Health] and said that I was worried about AIDS . . . [and thought] we ought to be doing something to make people aware of it.

These people, and others like them, proved to have been important catalysts for initiating action on HIV/AIDS within their health authorities. Some, indeed, went on to become key figures in the field, the 'product champions' (Stocking 1985) of the HIV/AIDS issue. As we shall see in a section devoted to them in a later chapter, these tended to be powerful people within the health authority and had particular personal characteristics, entrepreneurial skills and leadership qualities, which enabled them to play major roles in shaping the structure and content of service delivery.

However, not all the early 'prophets' were as well placed, or as temperamentally suited, to take a high profile lead on the issue. So we cannot see these characteristics as critical to the task of raising awareness. What they did all share, however, was what, in an earlier paper (Ferlie and Bennett 1992), we have described as a 'conversion' experience, a process of sometimes quite sudden recognition that HIV/AIDS was important and that they personally should do something about it.

Such conviction was vital because these prophets, like their biblical predecessors, often had to endure considerable scepticism, even from close colleagues: 'I can remember very much a feeling, and I'm sure he probably got it too, of 'He's off on his hobby horse again!'

However, they were not readily deterred by opposition. Thus, while not all prophets went on to become product champions, they showed some attributes similar to those of the successful entrepreneurs studied by Welsh and White (1981) in their persistence and determination to overcome hurdles and in being relatively impervious to short-term setbacks and failures.

Confirmed cases of HIV and AIDS

To a certain extent, of course, scepticism was understandable when, as in the provincial authorities, there were few if any patients during the early years of the epidemic. However, it proved just as difficult to convince some people in the London authorities, where a rapid buildup of cases occurred from 1983 onwards. There were rapid and unexpected mood shifts in these high prevalence localities:

> We could not get other people to take it seriously. We knew we were going to have real patients and real problems and people seemed to flip between not being bothered and not caring, and it was something minor and peripheral, to being something that was so serious that it was untouchable.
>
> (health service respondent)

The government did not seem to be taking the issue seriously either, and one respondent recalled the occasion when a member of staff argued on TV with the then Minister of Health in 1983 or 1984:

> Now at that time about fourteen or fifteen had been diagnosed or had died with AIDS, and he was saying, 'well, how many corpses do you need, do you need twenty, a hundred, two hundred, when is it enough? You can see what is happening in the States'.

Nevertheless, compared with having no patients at all, there can be no doubt that being able to prove the existence of either cases of AIDS or a substantial HIV-infected population did help to raise the profile of the issue within a health authority. This meant that another of the factors affecting whether or not an authority was early in reacting to HIV/AIDS was its geographical and population characteristics. The gay movement of the 1960s had led to London and certain provincial cities becoming particular centres for gay social life (Philips, 1988). One regional city, for instance, was described by a respondent as:

> A meeting place and social place for gay men backed up by the City Council's policy towards gay men and equal opportunities . . . a centre for gay people to both live in and travel to for their economic means and for a social meeting place.

People who inject drugs, and particularly young and disadvantaged drug users who may be most likely to share syringes (Local Authority Association 1988) also tend to be concentrated in cities, while people with haemophilia traditionally obtain most of their medical care from regional units, which, as noted earlier, are likely to be found in teaching authorities in major cities.

These factors combined meant that from early on a relatively small number of health authorities throughout the country *knew* they had considerable numbers of infected patients. In many of our authorities this had a key influence in raising awareness of the local relevance of the issue, mainly because of the reaction of staff, as discussed in the next section.

Staff anxieties

One way in which known cases of HIV or AIDS influenced awareness of the issue within the health authority was that it did not take long for staff, particularly in London, where most of the early cases were treated, to realize that there was a possibility of them coming into contact with infected patients.

Around 1983–84, media coverage of the epidemic was increasing, but still relatively little was known for certain about modes of transmission. In these circumstances, it was understandable that staff, particularly ancillary staff whose knowledge of medical matters was limited, were worried. Some groups took more extreme attitudes towards the need for protective clothing than others. In one London incident ambulance staff arrived in 'spacesuits' resulting in what was described by one respondent as 'a slanging match in front of the hospital'.

Outside London, where the buildup of AIDS cases was much slower, staff anxieties could be triggered solely by the media, as a respondent in one of our authorities recalled:

> The Government issued some green booklets with advice to people in general which I first heard about on breakfast television. There was Frank Bough waving this *Government Guidelines on AIDS* from the television set and I knew on that Friday morning there was going to be trouble at the hospital... the X-ray staff, the porters, the domestics, everybody was extremely worried.

This incident marked the beginning of a managerial response to HIV/ AIDS as an issue for the whole health authority, rather than relating solely to a few patients on a ward. Statements were issued to staff, the general manager started to ask questions about control of infection issues and a working party was convened to produce comprehensive guidelines for staff dealing with infected patients.

Similar processes, with the emphasis on instituting and improving procedures for ensuring the safety of staff, occurred in all our authorities around this period; partly provoked by expressed staff anxieties and partly by the Department of Health issuing health authorities with the first guidelines on AIDS from the Advisory Committee on Dangerous Pathogens.

Recognition of the wider relevance of the issue

Acknowledging HIV/AIDS as a control of infection issue for a health authority, however, was a long way from perceiving it as an issue that went beyond those narrow confines. Action was taken to tighten up standards and inform staff of such facts as were available, but the conceptual leap that would have allowed HIV/AIDS to have been seen as a strategic problem of major importance was still not made by most managers within health authorities. One general manager arriving in post in a high prevalence area as late as 1986 remembered: 'I don't recall it as an immediate problem, I think it certainly became a bigger issue as time went on, but when I first came here I don't recall it. Nobody said "this is the most important thing"'.

Even within specialist services it was possible for the significance of HIV/AIDS to go unrecognized:

> All we heard about at the very beginning was AIDS, and there was no panic on the part of drugs services at all . . . we actually started seeing clients in January 1986, we had no information whatsoever about HIV/AIDS at that time, and it was certainly at the earliest late that year that [information started coming through] and even then it was a very slow process and a gradual enlightenment. And then you suddenly thought 'God! What are we doing about all this? We need to be telling people about this.'
>
> (drugs services respondent)

The pervading lack of urgency amongst colleagues meant that many of those who were early in sensing the importance of the issue looked outside their own immediate circles for help and support in their mission. This eclecticism was demonstrated in the early *ad hoc* working groups on HIV/AIDS. These were notable for the inclusion of a very wide range of health service, local authority and voluntary sector representatives, unlike some of the later, more institutionalized, AIDS Action Groups (established in 1986 by official directive from the Department of Health).

The local social and political climate

The efforts of aware individuals to raise the profile of the issue could be helped or hindered by the local social and political climate. For instance, liberal attitudes towards minority groups tend to be characteristic of a university culture. This liberalism facilitated early health promotion efforts focused on the gay population in a number of authorities, as did a very radical political tradition in one Labour-dominated city council, where the battle for gay rights had been fought, and largely won, long before HIV/AIDS became an issue. In another city, however, the local authority, though also under Labour control, opposed gay organizations and greatly impeded early efforts to raise awareness, as a respondent described:

The problem, though, is AIDS being seen as a gay issue, and gays are perceived as being the looney left. There are Labour parties that are pro-gay and they are the looney left. [This city] is a middle of the road Labour party, therefore you can't have anything to do with AIDS, because AIDS is gay, which is looney left. So do nothing!

Social attitudes towards prevention initiatives involving such things as sex education in schools, particularly those with a strong religious tradition, also varied by locality: 'In [certain types of school] it becomes a very much more sensitive issue . . . they have been very reluctant to get anything like a sex education programme in operation' (health service respondent).

This loss of nerve was reinforced by new legislation making school governors directly responsible for the provision of sex education in schools, which was seen as sometimes leading to a more restrictive approach.

As difficult, or even more difficult, could be public and professional attitudes towards initiatives for injecting drug users. Following the relatively permissive 1960s, the national stance on drug use progressively hardened in the 1970s, though in some areas of Britain guidelines towards enforcement of the laws on possession were interpreted more rigorously than others. Injecting equipment was not readily available in many areas, and was often confiscated if found. This led to widespread sharing of needles, a highly efficient way of passing on blood-borne infections such as hepatitis and HIV.

The idea that clean syringes and needles should be made freely available in the interests of preventing spread of infection predated HIV, as Stimson et al. (1988) point out, but was highly politically controversial on grounds of public safety (discarded needles could cause injury): 'There is a danger of the whole thing getting closed down . . . we could reach the point where public pressure makes it almost impossible to continue if there are lots of needles found in the street.' It was also controversial on the moral grounds that it was likely to encourage and/or perpetuate illegal injecting and promote addiction. One respondent recalled a local politician blocking early plans for needle exchange because he saw 'the whole AIDS and drugs thing as dirty and sinful, as bad and wrong'. Raising awareness of HIV/AIDS was thus also affected by perceptions of the political acceptability of the issue, and the degree to which involvement might enhance or diminish personal standing: 'You can become an instant expert on AIDS by just standing still because everybody else steps backwards or walks away from it as fast as possible' (health service respondent). One Health Authority Chair spoke of 'crossing the barrier' when describing his struggle to come to terms with his fears about dealing with the subject, commenting: 'Even having a sticker in my car 'AIDS CONCERNS US ALL'; I've got my neighbours thinking 'Well! What's going on?' – as if it's something shocking.'

There could thus be an unease around HIV/AIDS, which, though largely unacknowledged could, and in some cases almost certainly did, inhibit the recognition process at organizational level.

Concluding discussion

We have seen that HIV arose during a period of increasing financial stringency and rapid structural and organizational change in the NHS, factors that were claiming much management attention and did not facilitate early recognition of a new health issue. However, despite the generally difficult financial situation, the relatively high status our case study authorities enjoyed implied somewhat more favourable climates for the endorsement and resourcing of new ventures.

As far as the 'official' health care system was concerned, interest in HIV/AIDS was at first limited to a few specialist researchers, and although medical professionals, particularly in the clinical specialties likely to become involved in caring for patients, gradually became aware of the issue, individual clinicians varied in the degree to which they perceived its wider importance and local relevance. SMOs also played an important role in stimulating awareness, although these groups were best developed in London and the major regional centres. Although vocal, these organizations had a patchy effect on the statutory system at the level of local policy making, and their influence on local authorities tended to depend on the local political climate.

Within the NHS, awareness of HIV as a strategic issue tended to be promoted by a few key people, often, but not always, clinicians, who, for particular and idiosyncratic reasons, sensed the significance and urgency of the issue early and took a personal interest. Even within the same hospital, clinicians varied in the stance that they took towards the new issue. In one of our cases, a small, key, group were convinced by 1981–82 that a major problem was about to break, using analysis (access to data) but also intuition. The presence of patients, either with AIDS or HIV-infected, was not always a necessary precondition for raising awareness, though where there were confirmed cases, requests for resources were more likely to succeed. Also, where patients with AIDS were being nursed, recognition of the need to make some organizational response to the issue often came about through staff anxieties about the dangers of cross-infection. Where there were few actual cases, concern about the future could be effective in raising awareness if there was seen to be a substantial 'at risk' population within the authority, because of existing patterns of drug use, travel and migration within urban areas, and as a result of local social and political attitudes to minority groups.

The speed with which HIV/AIDS triggered an organizational response was also affected by the local social and political climate. A history of cooperation on health issues between health and the local authority facilitated early joint initiatives, as did liberal attitudes towards minority groups. On the other hand, in some cases early attempts to raise awareness of HIV foundered because of local public or professional opposition to initiatives aimed at drug users or updating sex education.

Are there generalizable lessons?

In some ways, of course, HIV/AIDS is an exceptional case. The appearance in the organizational environment of a major new issue that is qualitatively different from anything previously experienced must be a comparatively rare event for any organization. On the other hand, it might have been expected that its very novelty would have led to early recognition and take-up. Instead of which, as we have seen, not all organizations made an immediate response to the issue, and in those where reaction was relatively early, the response came mostly from a few particular individuals who were earlier than their contemporaries in sensing the issue and recognizing its importance.

Johnson and Scholes (1984) suggest that a number of factors accumulate in the issue recognition process, ultimately forcing recognition of a problem at organizational level. This seems to be borne out in our cases, though different factors were important in different authorities. Huczynski and Buchanan (1991) differentiate between pressure exerted by environmental factors, either internal or external to the organization, and that resulting from proactive measures taken by managers anticipating change. Looking at our data, we can see that the prime external factor was the identification of HIV/AIDS, but that other external factors, such as local population characteristics and relations with other statutory and non-statutory organizations also played a part. Internal factors such as a 'scientific culture', the strength of local SMOs and the presence or absence of specialist facilities also affected the process of recognition, as did the proactive thinking of a small group of people who sensed the issue in advance of any environmental pressure to respond.

Thus far, it seems that the process of recognition of HIV/AIDS demonstrates that broadly similar mechanisms were involved to those which operate for any new issue within organizations. However, this broad framework gives considerable latitude for variation, and the literature frequently fails to mention, much less explain, the reasons for the differential responses made by organizations to the same trigger factors. It may be, therefore, that what we have to consider is not so much the triggers themselves, but a linking concept of 'situational relevance'. In other words, that there were particular situations in our health authorities that made HIV/AIDS fit in with, rather than be contrary to, the needs of the moment.

It may be that psychological theories of information processing and selective attention have something to offer here. There is experimental evidence (for a review see Fitts and Posner 1973: Chapter 4) to suggest that individuals whose attention is focused on one set of stimuli cannot efficiently process another set of stimuli simultaneously. For instance, it is possible to listen to one speaker and understand and remember what is being said, while simultaneously ignoring and having no memory of the content of another speech delivered at the same volume. However, if there is something about the stimulus that is not being attended to and which is particularly relevant to the individual, such as their own name being mentioned by the speaker they are ignoring, this is likely to engage their attention (Cherry 1953).

It seems possible that the process of recognition of the HIV/AIDS issue in our early-responding health authorities occurred as a result of a similar sort of mechanism, with the issue attracting attention because it was relevant to the particular situations, either of individuals or of an aspect or aspects of their organization, whereas in other health authorities these particular circumstances did not apply.

The process of issue recognition we have traced in this chapter suggests that a number of different factors were important in raising awareness of HIV/AIDS, but that their influence was not either discrete or simultaneous, but additive over time. As we have seen, even before AIDS was identified, there were both internal and external factors in each of our case study authorities that might have suggested that they were likely to be relatively receptive to a new health issue (comparatively good resourcing, scientific organizational culture, for instance); and other factors that would have enabled us to argue exactly the opposite (general financial stringency, dense management agenda). The theme of differential receptivity to organizational change, and specifically the suggestion that particularly receptive contexts for change can be identified, has been recently reviewed and discussed by Pettigrew et al. (1992). However, receptivity implies a degree of passivity, an openness and readiness to external forces for change. The concept of 'situational relevance' complements and extends this by adding a dynamic element arising from individual or collective cognition, which may explain why similar environmental influences, when applied to similarly receptive contexts, may or may not 'trigger' a change process.

In Chapter 6, which is concerned with early service development in our case study authorities, we explore the effects of this cognitive aspect of the change process by considering how different groups of people, having recognized that HIV/AIDS was relevant to their situation, set about the process of persuading others of the need to take action on the issue.

Note

1 Morbidity and Mortality Weekly Report, published by the Centers for Disease Control, Atlanta.

6

Moving into action – rising concern and crisis

Introduction

We now move on to look at how the new HIV/AIDS issue was constructed as a legitimate focus for activity by the health care organizations studied. This stage immediately followed the recognition by at least some people that this issue now existed (as was explored in the last chapter). The problem that was emerging had thus been sensed (1982–85), but a formal organizational response not yet provided.

This next phase (say Spring 1985 to Autumn 1986) can be designated as an early period of organizational response to the HIV/AIDS issue, being characterized by generally rising levels of concern. This led to a pattern of individual initiatives, *ad hoc* development, the formation of small groups and the release of some small-scale resources. Of course, there were also powerful sources of resistance to the issue in many of the organizations studied, and as yet nothing substantial in the way of formal structures, national recognition or support was evident.

We see this stage as coming to an end in late 1986, when there was an explosion of media interest, when national policy on HIV/AIDS began to take shape, when progressively generous finance was made available and when formal structures were instituted to implement guidelines. At this stage, a crisis mentality was increasingly evident, peaking in Spring 1987. Throughout this period, incipient service systems were developing very rapidly as resources and political attention increased.

We may be able to draw some parallels here with processes evident in Pettigrew's (1985) study of how managers effect change in a large and complex private sector organization, namely ICI. ICI experienced a business 'crisis' in 1979–81, which was utilized as a lever by those who wanted to achieve a fundamental strategic redirection. Some individual actors had sensed this problem in an earlier period, but were unable at that stage to get their ideas for change accepted.

From a political process point of view, Pettigrew argued that it was important not to rush prematurely from problem sensing to action, as actions recommended about problems that themselves are not seen as legitimate may lead to the rejection of the change idea. So individual problem sensing should be accompanied by building a more shared appreciation. Initially the concern may be voiced by a single visionary change leader, a deviant or a heretic, sensing and imprecisely articulating a critical performance gap, but:

> The key management task here is to more broadly educate the organization by building on the perspective, information, and contacts of the early adopters. In effect to recognize the group doing this early sensing, to broaden the group by helping to connect them to peers, bosses, and subordinates with similar views and to prepare more of a critical mass of people to help influence key power figures.
>
> (Pettigrew 1985: 474)

Pettigrew suggests that in this second phase of generating a broader acknowledgement and concern with the problem, an important management of change task is to help the very early adopters and any supportive power figures to maintain and develop a structured dialogue about the problem. This should not be seen as a unilinear process, but one that is emergent, and as such characterized by iterations, dead ends, and sudden spurts of movement. We can see some parallels here with HIV/AIDS. For example, early visionaries in one Inner London hospital were active in proclaiming the importance of the issue from 1982 onwards. Yet, as late as 1984, there was little evidence of gathering momentum as the locus of managerial responsibility for the issue remained unclear and little planning was taking place. When asked how much time managers spent on the AIDS issue in 1984, one respondent replied:

> Very little. Really very little. I mean it would have been one of those issues I am sure where we would have said 'Yes, it is a problem, and we know we have got to put more money into it' and I can't even remember what we did put into it, I just know we did increase nurses.

We shall return to this argument in the concluding section when we compare our analysis of strategic change in this rather different setting with that of Pettigrew. Here we argue that the securing of early activity around HIV/AIDS was achieved through a number of mechanisms. These mechanisms can be seen as exhibiting a roughly temporal progression as follows:

- Concern and lobbying from SMOs;
- Action from individual clinical 'product champions';
- The launching of central initiatives and provision of special resources;
- The appointment of specialist staff;
- The involvement of professional and managerial groups;
- The mobilizing effect of a perceived crisis.

Concern and lobbying from social movement organizations

As of early 1986, voluntary organizations concerned about AIDS (such as the AIDS Forum) in [the District] began to mushroom. The AIDS Forum organized a Conference and booked a room that would hold 500, but in the end some 2500 turned up. But there was some feeling also that such organizations were difficult to sustain and could quickly go from boom to bust.

(researcher's analysis in a primary case study)

Nationally and at a local level, social movements and SMOs played an important role in the development of the strategic response to HIV/AIDS and were often the first bodies to display concern (from 1982–83 onwards). Not only did they act as direct service providers themselves, supporting those ill with HIV-related symptoms through their 'buddying' network and supplying information and advice on prevention of infection through telephone helplines, but they also lobbied the statutory sector to move the HIV/AIDS issue further up the 'official' agenda.

As already discussed in Chapter 3, SMOs may display organizational forms that are very different from formally value-neutral bureaucracies. SMOs are held together less by hierarchical or contractual relationships and more by a strong culture or a shared ideology. There may be strong swings within these settings from periods of high enthusiasm and activity to periods of withdrawal and apathy, resulting in a high turnover of personnel.

Where HIV/AIDS is concerned, most of the early initiatives outside the medical profession came from activists in the gay community, and from people involved in 'alternative' rather than traditional approaches to medicine, which emphasized non-standard patient involvement in therapy. In terms of approaches to health education, these models could lead to a preference for 'experiential' training models (i.e. consciousness raising) over more traditional didactic approaches.

Such social movements had been particularly influential in three of the localities studied. Perhaps surprisingly, these were all in regional centres rather than Inner London, where the dominance of the teaching hospital was strongest. Here we give two contrasting examples.

A radical social movement tradition

The role of the gay movement was particularly apparent in one regional centre, where it played a dominant role in service development during the early years. The initial activity undertaken in this, as in many places, was the formation of a telephone helpline. This then became a focus for political activism, counselling and direct service provision, including befriending and outreach work to various groups, such as drug users. However, this list of activities is not so very different from those undertaken, or at any rate planned, by the gay movement in some of our other cases, so we need to ask just why the movement developed to be not simply successful, but to take a much stronger lead role in policy making and planning than similar movements elsewhere.

One explanation for this is that, as pointed out by Eckstein (1960), an important determinant of the form of action taken by pressure groups is whether other interest groups in their environments favour a high key or low key approach. In this particular case, the very high political profile taken by the voluntary sector received active support and cooperation from the local medical product champion, a community physician, and other members of the department who had a radical approach to public health and emphasized the importance of consumer involvement. Support also came from a left wing Labour Council. In addition, the case being put forward by this coalition of interest was strengthened by a highly publicized incident in 1985 when a person with AIDS was detained in hospital under the recently revised Public Health (Infectious Diseases) Act. This caused a furore about civil rights, which deeply embarrassed the statutory sector, and ensured that the interests of the voluntary sector received even more attention.

A liberal social movement tradition

This situation can be contrasted with that obtaining where the dominant culture affecting social movements was essentially a liberal one. Within one such health authority – based on a powerful university – an atmosphere of cooperation and shared responsibility existed, but it was clear, none the less, that the true power over decision making and resources remained with the statutory sector, a situation that was challenged without real success by some of the more radically minded members of the gay movement:

> [the gay movement's helpline] ... is an organization of very well
> meaning people who are for the most part out of sight or removed,

you know, they are doing this because it is something good to do
... actually they found [X] and me very hard work, because we were
saying, 'Look, there are so many things we could be doing, we could
be doing education, we could be doing this or that' – a more activist
approach.

In this authority, norms of politeness and of acceptable conduct acted
to reduce the potential pay-off from any overt challenge. In contrast to the
situation in the previous example, where people were used to comba-
tive relationships, confrontation was not seen as a way in which civilized
people should behave.

The SMOs observed, therefore, exhibited rather different styles, perhaps
influenced by the host organizational and political culture. As we explored
in Chapter 4, some of the literature suggests that SMOs are unlikely to
be effective in intervening in formal decision making processes, given the
danger of sectarianism and of withdrawal from the wider world. On the
whole, this scenario, at least in organizational terms (although individual
attitudes could be rigid), was not apparent in our sample. However, although Downs' (1967) concept of 'zealotry' is probably too extreme to be
applied in its entirety to most organizations studied, there was some evidence of groups becoming fixated on particular ways of addressing issues
such as health promotion, despite evidence that they were not in fact being
effective, and after receiving suggestions for alternative approaches.

At national level, of course, the Terrence Higgins Trust and other gay
groups had been very early movers in mobilizing support for their perspective on the HIV/AIDS issue. Many of their ideas, such as the importance
of confidentiality and the need for counselling, were legitimated by government approval very early on, putting them at an advantage *vis-à-vis* other
groups who might otherwise have been expected to marginalize them. As
soon as patients began to arrive, a number of these SMOs were effective
in constructing an alliance with early clinical product champions (see next
section) at ward and clinic level.

Agents of change: the clinical 'product champions'

From 1983 onwards there was a speedy building up of service systems
around those clinicians early in the field, demonstrating the early stages
of a process lifecycle which has been described in many other settings (Easton and Rothschild 1987) and is characterized by rapid developmental
change and lack of standardization.

The 'product champion' has been found to be an important element of
the innovation process in both industrial (Rothwell 1976) and health care
settings (Stocking 1985). There is now also the beginnings of a literature
on product champions in organizational process: a product champion

(Burgelman and Sayles 1986) is seen as being able to work effectively in a non-programmed environment. HIV/AIDS was certainly uncharted territory and those early in the field needed not only to be aware of their own need to acquire knowledge, but also to have the ability to create from the little that was known some way of moving forward. The following quotation from a doctor identified as a key clinical product champion in one of the case study authorities encapsulates this view of the role: 'Somebody who wants to learn but can also see their way through the morass and see a direction, a certain vision of what needs to be achieved.'

Another attribute of the product champion, suggest Burgelman and Sayles (1986), is the ability to deal with a variety of groups over which there is no formal control, each of which may have different or contradictory goals and each of which is critical to project success. This raises the question of diplomatic skills and of coalition building. The effective product champion (Rothwell and Zegweld 1982) may also need considerable power and prestige in order to influence the informal politics of organizational decision making.

In Chapter 5 we saw the emergence of 'prophets' – the early sensors of a new and potentially very important issue. They were instrumental in raising awareness, but not all went on to become true 'product champions' for the HIV/AIDS issue. To become a product champion it was not only necessary to have vision, but to have the potential capacity to drive forward proposals for service development. Within the NHS, this meant doctors, mostly clinical consultants in the key specialties (see Chapter 3), but also some influential public health physicians. What is interesting here is that although, as noted earlier, these were low status specialties, the individual characteristics of the champions enabled them to overcome this disadvantage and exert enormous influence on their organizations and at national level, long before the issue was officially recognized by government.

What were these characteristics, which set the champions apart from other colleagues in the same specialties who, despite access to the same information, did not respond, and indeed were often dismissive of the very idea of HIV/AIDS having any relevance to their future practice? Though they were very different as individuals, they all had in common a belief in the crucial importance of HIV/AIDS, an enthusiasm for promoting greater awareness and interest in the issue, and a broad view of its relevance outside the narrow confines of medical practice.

Some people had a particular personal interest in the issue, but often it seemed to be a question of having been in a particular place at a particular time. The early clinical champions often made a personal and 'unofficial' decision to move into the emerging HIV/AIDS field, using their personal ability to win 'soft money' (e.g. research grants) to get incipient service systems up and running. By the time management realized what was going on, it was sometimes too late to control the inbuilt pressure for further expansion.

The early clinical product champions also showed a most unusual degree of eclecticism, given the traditional reluctance of professionals to share their expertise with others. In part, this reflected the pervading lack of knowledge about the disease during the first few years. There *were* no experts, and this opened the way for the sort of dialogue with patients about their treatment and care needs that would have been unthinkable in more established settings. In this situation, key clinicians often rapidly shed outdated attitudes and became recognized by patients as providing a quality service:

> [Doctor X] has moved miles in his approach to patients. He integrates all the best facets of the voluntary sector . . . with the patient being involved in the care and respecting what the patient wants to do, and he is tremendous now, much further ahead than any of his colleagues because of working in this field.
>
> (voluntary sector respondent)

Responding to patient pressure in this way should not be seen, however, as a total transfer of professional power to other groups. This was essentially a process of high status people 'giving away' power in one direction, patient-centred services, in order to keep it in another by remaining the focus of service provision. This has been a key characteristic of the development of HIV/AIDS services, and has contributed to the centralization of services in specialist acute sector settings.

Another aspect of the eclecticism of the early product champions was demonstrated in the formation of early *ad hoc* working groups on HIV/AIDS. These were notable for the inclusion of different medical specialties and local authority and voluntary sector representatives, and a great contrast to the usual medically dominated structure of advisory groups on clinical issues. In part their multidisciplinary character was undoubtedly due to the lack of widespread interest in HIV/AIDS within the specialties at that time and the determination of the voluntary sector lobby to be included, but there was also evident a vision amongst key clinicians of an appropriate future development for services.

This sense of vision, so characteristic of entrepreneurs of all kinds as they seek to attain, not only change, but a new concept (Mintzberg 1989), resulted in a determination to develop the kinds of services the champions felt were needed, regardless of even the most protracted opposition, and some were prepared to use every means at their disposal to manipulate the situation: 'I recognized early on that the only way we'd get [funders] to move was to embarrass them, and . . . we got onto the newspapers and the box and turned the temperature up and got them to respond' (clinical product champion).

Coalition building

As the last quotation suggests, product champions also varied in their diplomatic skills. Putting together a wider base was of critical importance, but although most product champions in our sample had a degree of personal status, this did not necessarily mean that they were the most powerful people in their environments. The approach taken to coalition building varied considerably according to personal style and preferences. Some wanted broad influence, others to build services under their direct control. Contrast these two approaches:

> That really has been my role, to see that each of those groups has its target. To see first of all that the target is recognized and that people are moving on those targets in a coordinated fashion . . . that they have the right information, see that they know who to ask for medical support when they need it, see that they actually do think critically about what they are trying to do, and also to make sure that they work as far as they can with other people and do not clash with those people.

> People know me by now, that if I say that I'm going to do something and I've got the money to do it, then they are not going to stop me. You know, it is a question of, they can decide to be on my side or not, and it's probably better for them if they are on my side.

For some, 'managing up' was an important aspect of diplomatic activity:

> I think I am probably the only physician in the District who has actually made a point of developing as good a relationship as quickly as one can with new ministers . . . even though in a sense one is working with managers here, there is always the time when you feel that if they are really going to syphon off the money and play silly buggers, then one has to off side them, and you can only off side them by going very much higher, and I think that is important, that they know that that is a rule of the game, but that one would not do it . . .

'Managing across' was rather more common, with early champions of HIV/AIDS gathering around them other important people who could help to further their cause. In one health authority, the original product champion, a consultant in genitourinary medicine, was particularly fortunate in recruiting another comrade at arms, a community medicine specialist, at an early stage. The energy and enthusiasm of the two together proved irresistible, and despite having very few patients, the authority forged ahead, making alliances with the city council and the voluntary sector on the way, and developing structures and making key appointments to work in the field long before anything similar was suggested at national level.

In another health authority, the product champion built up even broader alliances with key acute medical specialists and general management, and set up a research team within his own department working on a range of topics from the basic science to sociological and behavioural aspects of the epidemic. An important change in the cast of actors in this authority took place in 1984 when the professor of medicine (a general physician with an interest in thoracic medicine) made a decision to declare an interest in AIDS work. A focus now began to emerge for inpatient work, which was seen as clinically highly appropriate because of the frequent presentation of patients with pneumonia, and while such diversification also helped the product champion maintain his bed state, which might otherwise be under threat, the presence of a powerful and well respected friend within the mainstream acute specialties certainly helped the traditionally more marginal genitourinary physicians to argue a case.

Not all authorities saw quite so much coalition building as this in the early years. Much depended, as we have already suggested, on the personal management style of the product champions. Organization theorists have identified a number of different types of coalition (Morgan 1986). The type most frequently found in our sample was a simple coalition of interest. Diverse people, often with different fundamental beliefs and values, agreeing to work together towards a common goal, in this case the development of services for HIV/AIDS.

However, collaboration could be brought about by the use of more political tactics. In one of our authorities part of the object was to consolidate the powerbase of the key actor. The following account describes the method used to call a meeting of people from different organizations to develop a joint strategy for HIV/AIDS. The convener, the local product champion, asked each nominee to forward information on the actions they had already taken on the issue, although he was by no means certain that everyone he was inviting was currently active in the field:

> ... they now had a problem, nobody was going to turn up at this meeting saying, 'We haven't done anything'. So that got an enormous flurry of activity going. Boom! Suddenly everyone was in action ... So they all turned up having done something ... it was then no longer possible to defend inaction, because there was a forum in which you had to turn up and defend it.

By taking the initiative in this way, and by offering himself to chair, and his organization to service, the resulting structure, the product champion ensured that he maintained and strengthened his position as the key figure on HIV/AIDS in the area.

Yet another way in which coalitions may be formed is through shared ideologies. Many of the voluntary organizations we studied subscribed to radical traditions, manifesting themselves in a concern for individual rights, and a belief in eradication of inequalities and in patient power. The style tended to be confrontational:

> If you have got a group of patients they can form a counterweight to the doctor's authority. [The consultant] was really threatened about that when this latest group started . . . and called [X] in and was very angry . . . I mean it is all about power and control of patients, and it is a very old-fashioned story.
>
> (voluntary sector respondent)

However, where such views were shared amongst many of the key actors in both the statutory and voluntary sector, as in the next example, this proved to be a particularly successful form of coalition, in terms of achieving its particular goals and objectives:

> I remember great arguments, but thinking back, we were extremely progressive to have the client group in . . . you realize how much we have come on in that they do allow the client to choose, and they do discuss as an equal, and for the first time in medicine this field is leading the way . . . certainly the client knows best, instead of the nurses and doctors.

Critical functions of the product champion role

In other places, clinical product champions ended up being the people who asked the difficult questions of management:

> The fact that the people who were put in a high managerial position in AIDS had no feel for, no instinctive view, let alone mental view of the issues, is a reflection on the fact that management intrinsically prefers to keep its distance and likes to cast the clinicians in the role of shroud wavers, and the difficult characters and the people who do not understand money.
>
> (clinical product champion)

The decision to come forward as an AIDS 'product champion' was not an easy one and could have far-reaching consequences, transforming the pace of work and long-term careers, for better or for worse. The glare of publicity could have negative as well as positive consequences if a perception grew of the product champion as only a 'media doctor.' Some innovators were in essence 'climbers' (Downs, 1967). HIV/AIDS, a high profile issue, with no organizational history behind it, and money available for new development, was custom-made for those at the beginning of their careers who were hoping to make their mark early: 'At that time it suddenly became a big thing, and [people] then realized it was a good thing to be in infectious diseases as this was a disease that was going somewhere.'

Some of these quickly moved onto successor issues. This was only one subgroup, though, and many others have stayed firmly committed to the field. On the negative side, some people found that they tended to be 'typecast' by AIDS, and that this had an adverse effect on prospects for working in other areas. Self-confidence and personality were other factors, as AIDS services tended to attract risk takers:

> I think personality has a lot to do with it in terms of being someone who is willing to play a few new games, learn a few new tricks ... AIDS attracted a lot of new people who came in to care for AIDS and they were people who were prepared to face the new and the unknown.
>
> (clinical product champion)

The picture of the product champion that emerges from our data, then, is not as homogeneous as one might have thought. There were clearly identifiable focal figures driving service development in all our health authorities but some managed without much status, particularly in the early days, although there was here a requirement to access other power centres. Some but not all had experienced a 'road to Damascus' conversion leading to their championing AIDS as a cause to the exclusion of all other concerns. There were some 'diplomats', but they were balanced by some whose ability to alienate the very people they wished to influence was legendary. What they all had, however, was a quality that Peters and Waterman (1982) identified as a key attribute of the champion – the ability to take responsibility for converting ideas into action. Our champions were the doers. They set up the *ad hoc* committees, they went ahead with getting people together and telling them about AIDS, they set up services on shoestrings by bending existing services to fit (often without waiting for permission), and they were prepared to work longer and harder than almost anyone else to achieve their goals.

Early central initiatives and resources

In the very early days, the first product champions used all sorts of devices to scrape together funds from different sources to get projects off the ground. Often the only way was to try to access 'soft' money by convincing someone of the need for research, a process memorably described by one respondent as: 'like carving money out of living rock'. However, with the advent of testing for HIV/AIDS in 1984–85, and also with the first results of cohort studies, it was becoming clear that there was a substantial pool of infection, most notably in Inner London but also in some regional centres.

Central government was also being heavily lobbied on the HIV/AIDS issue by key clinicians and, by late 1985, small special allocations were being made available by the Department of Health to high prevalence localities in Inner London. Small-scale as they were, these early allocations were nevertheless important in getting the localities started, following a period of organizational inertia in 1983–84. However, apart from some specific 'one-off' allocations for counselling and drugs services, and some capital funds for specialist units, until 1988, when the first ring-fenced monies were received, health authorities outside London were dependent for service development on money squeezed out of general funds. Unsurprisingly, much, if not all, of the decision-making around service development was mediated by this, and it was here that the entrepreneurial characteristics of some product champions came very much to the fore:

> I had a post due in the annual programme . . . it takes eighteen months to actually get someone in post through the annual programme mechanism . . . a post which was a health visitor equivalent, a sort of infectious disease liaison leg worker, because I felt we didn't really have enough bods on the ground to be contact tracing. And as the clock ran, as it were, to the point where we could actually spend the money I was increasingly saying to people 'Most of the interest in infectious disease posts will have to go into AIDS prevention so although it's an infectious disease post we ought perhaps just to look for someone who would be very useful to AIDS'.

However, for the many health authorities where early recognition of the HIV/AIDS issue had not occurred, and where no 'product champions' had emerged, lack of specific resources for service development undoubtedly tipped the balance in favour of doing nothing until the issue rose to prominence and government directives stimulated action.

Nevertheless, central government was supporting a number of service initiatives in the 1985–87 period: the provision of diagnostic facilities, ensuring safe blood transfusion facilities and the provision of counselling support; in addition, mostly through the efforts of the voluntary sector, some charity monies were coming onstream. Where service development had already started, the early movers were well placed to take advantage. However, even with money available, if a health authority or specialty lacked the necessary know-how to bid for it, opportunities could be lost.

For example, staff at the haemophilia centre in one of our authorities were struggling to support a large number of infected patients. They had never been in the frontline of the kind of battles for funding that doctors in more esoteric specialties, such as transplantation surgery, were used to. They simply assumed their problem was self-evident: 'We'd been asking . . . and, rather naïvely probably, thought we would get something, but didn't'. This particular staff team quickly learned not to be backward in coming forward, and before long they had mobilized some help from their local haemophilia society and were rattling government ministers' doors to substantial effect.

The appointment of specialist staff

With the advent of increasing sums of central money, specialist posts and teams began to emerge at local level, typically characterized by an energetic and campaigning style. They were sometimes appointed by the early clinical product champions, who wanted more of a focus for HIV/AIDS work, but were too busy themselves.

Often such staff should be seen as 'bureaucratic insurgents', moving from a voluntary sector background into a public sector setting. A key question was how specialists managed their boundaries with the wider organization, much of which might not share their relatively narrow interests. Nevertheless, they acted as a key focus for service development, not least because 'AIDS' in their job titles served as a signal that this was, at last, a legitimate issue.

Coordinator posts

HIV/AIDS coordinators emerged in a number of localities. In one regional centre studied, a very early appointment was made of an AIDS Liaison Officer, making headlines in the national press. This first post was quickly followed by other dedicated appointments, often focusing on prevention and health education.

The nature of the issue and the type and amount of resourcing available combined to attract applicants with particular personal characteristics. Appointments were temporary and salaries relatively low. Those applying for early posts were frequently young, bright, enthusiastic and with a background of activity in the voluntary sector.

The early generation of HIV/AIDS workers made a big impact on the statutory organizations in which they were employed. As, by all ordinary indicators (e.g. hierarchical status, span of control, even possession of expertise), they were relatively junior, we need to ask why this was so. One key factor was that they had powerful allies, being appointed for the most part by powerful patrons who both protected them and gave them autonomy. Second, their job titles often included words such as 'coordinator', 'facilitator' or 'liaison', which invested them with the power to cross boundaries and mediate between interest groups. They were also able to give their full time and attention to HIV/AIDS, which earlier advocates had often not been able to do.

On the other hand, as the field was developing rapidly, their newly acquired skills were at a premium and there tended to be a high turnover of staff. In addition, the very attributes (i.e. creativity and enthusiasm), which had quickly enabled them to make their mark in service development, were not often matched by the stamina required to carry on with routine and repetitive health promotion work. The main problem lay not in establishing successful programmes but in maintaining them. A further problem concerns status. Early appointments were high profile and supported by powerful sponsors in the medical product champions. Improvements in the financial situation and government support for coordinator posts focusing particularly on aspects of prevention and health education have led to appointments being made in most health authorities. Many post holders are now working in authorities where there are still no key medical champions for the issue. Now individual workers with no status of their own and lacking powerful sponsors may to lack profile and influence with senior management.

Special teams

In some localities, the HIV/AIDS issue was captured by a special team, financed through the special central allocation. This was perhaps easier in low prevalence localities where the acute sector had not yet developed a major interest in the issue, and where activity focused on preventive work.

One such project was sanctioned by the local health authority in autumn 1986. The first project manager took up post in May 1987, with a number of project workers starting that Autumn. It was seen as a high profile response to the challenge of HIV/AIDS in an authority that was still seen as low prevalence, hence the emphasis on health prevention activity. The project went on to develop in a number of innovative and interesting ways.

A major issue concerns the management of the boundary between the special project and other services. In this case, links with other public services which shared similar values as the team (e.g. the youth service) were good, although those with gay groups were not as extensive as might have been expected. However links with other groupings, which displayed different value systems (e.g. police, senior management, private employers), seemed weaker.

The involvement of professional and managerial groups

The public health function

In many of the most active authorities, the public health function played an influential and shaping role in the legitimation of early activity. The HIV/AIDS issue was generally seen as a key and rightful task for public health medicine to pick up. This early role became further institutionalized as national guidance emerged in 1986 which required health authorities to set up more formal structures, often based on a public health consultant as the nominated physician.

Their structural importance reflected the earlier tendency to interpret the issue as one requiring professional public health and epidemiological expertise (Fox et al. 1989). The issue, after all, took the form of an epidemic and as such could be seen as a core part of the public health remit. At national level, the Chief Medical Officer (Sir Donald Acheson) similarly acted as a major focus for policy making.

Sometimes public health physicians took a broadly based interest in HIV/AIDS policy issues across the range of specialties, thus helping to combat parochialism and isolation. Against that the function itself was patchily developed (Cm 289, 1988), sometimes fairly marginal, and in places losing ground in the face of the new general management.

Although public health played a role in all our health authorities in this time period, two rather different responses can be discerned. In most localities, the public health physician effectively acted to 'hold the ring', perhaps coordinating the response but not taking a central role in service innovation and development. In a smaller number of cases, public health physicians were already taking a more central role, often displaying a great interest in prevention initiatives, evaluation and working with affected communities and SMOs. Here the public health clinicians might also act as an important bridge into direct liaison with affected communities. However, in only a minority of instances were the key product champions drawn from public health.

While in most cases, public health was clearly recognized as appropriately taking a lead role, in some of the authorities, there were signs of a struggle for control of the HIV/AIDS issue between public health on the one hand and general management on the other. There could also be problems if, as in some cases, the nominated physician had little interest in the issue. In such circumstances their AIDS Action Committees tended to be less than effective.

The role of general management

Appointments were being made to new general management posts in 1985–86. How did these newly appointed managers react to the emergent HIV/AIDS issue? Their agendas dominated by questions of financial control, the new general managers were on the whole dull in their response to HIV/AIDS. As one respondent remarked: 'general managers are not turned on by AIDS, but by the tag that attaches to AIDS'. Indeed, another respondent was developing a financial model of general managerial behaviour: what was the point beyond which the special financial allocation had to rise before general managers would start to attend meetings?

Giving the HIV/AIDS issue to a general manager who lacked a sense of personal ownership was counterproductive and could lead to a damping down of the whole management process. Nor – on the whole – was there much evidence of conscious utilization of the HIV/AIDS issue as a containable testbed for a more general organizational development brief.

There were some important redeeming features and interesting exceptions. Those managers who developed the greatest interest in HIV/AIDS tended to be concentrated in the areas of highest prevalence, perhaps involved in the policy process nationally, perhaps drawn from clinical backgrounds or perhaps interested in a lateral and creative way. Here is an example of active and interested management from Inner London. In one site, a newly appointed District General Manager had been keeping a watching brief:

> The funny thing was that AIDS had not impinged on my consciousness at all until I got the job here . . . I became aware that (a) there was such a thing as AIDS and (b) [the locality] was in the thick of it. And then I got here, it went WROOM! From that moment on, more and more time was taken up. I sat [on the key committee] just to get the hang of it, and very swiftly a District ethic that AIDS is important takes over.

The District General Manager was here intervening managerially in the AIDS issue from late 1986 onwards.

The mobilizing role of crisis

Dutton (1987) has argued that the processing of strategic issues will be very different in crisis and non-crisis situations. Certainly, in 1986 and 1987, the HIV/AIDS issue nationally attracted a 'crisis' label with unprecedented advertising campaigns and media coverage. The early epidemiology was taken as indicating that Britain was only four years or so behind the explosive US epidemic (in fact the pace of the epidemic grew far more slowly). The issue characteristics used by Dutton to define a crisis (importance, immediacy and uncertainty) all applied to the HIV issue, indeed it was said that there had been nothing like it in health care since the Second World War.

Alongside the national AIDS crisis, particular localities were experiencing their own local crises. There was the discovery, for instance, that many haemophiliac patients had been infected through receiving contaminated Factor VIII. One local product champion used this to 'construct' a local crisis around HIV/AIDS:

> Because of the way that the haemophiliacs had been infected our figures looked worse than they really were . . . We had an extra

hundred infected people in the stats that were part of a different epidemic that had peaked, because 60 per cent of the haemophiliacs had been infected and not any more of them . . . It made it look as if we had more . . . and assuming doubling times and all that you get to horrendous numbers quite quickly. So, in other words, we had anxiety levels out of all proportion to the numbers.

In another health authority, a local crisis arose literally overnight when a virologist, practising the new HTLV-3 test on stored blood sera from drug users, quite unexpectedly discovered that 38 per cent tested positive:

> We went to bed on Tuesday evening believing that whatever [the health authority's] AIDS problem was, it was likely to be no better and no worse than anyone else's, and we got up on Wednesday morning and found that we had this huge number of infected people.
>
> (health service respondent)

However, a 'crisis' did not emerge in every locality, despite the national triggers, because in some areas the caseload was too low, or because there had been prior recent experience of dealing with an epidemic. In one case, for instance there had been a local outbreak of tuberculosis and lessons gained from managing this provided an important coping mechanism.

The data collected leads us to propose a three-phase model to explain organizational behaviour when confronted with an issue perceived as posing a long-term threat to the familiar assumptions and working practices on which an organization is based. The model bears some resemblance to psychological theories about the effect on individual performance of the degree of arousal in response to a stimulus. These suggest that experiencing the same stimulus at varying degrees of intensity may produce differing levels of performance, with higher levels of arousal associated with increased energy and improved performance (Hebb 1955), but that very high levels of arousal, leading to fear and anxiety about the possibility of making an appropriate response, may lead to paralysis rather than appropriate action (Tyhurst 1951).

Thus as we have already argued, in many areas there was initially a destabilizing crisis of anxiety in line with the 'epidemic psychology' model (Strong 1990). In the short term, the issue was often characterized by 'incidents', waves of panic and fear, and staff refusal to work with patients.

In the medium term, as anxiety subsided to what might be seen as approaching a more 'optimal' level, the perception of a local crisis often had energizing and creative effects, leading to an outburst of enthusiasm and activity. Ideas for new services were being generated and implemented, resources were being obtained and qualitatively different care regimes being introduced where patients could have greater control over treatment (e.g.

user representation on drug trial committees). Unlike other more intractable issues in the NHS, rapid change seemed possible.

Increasingly, once the first sense of panic had subsided, an important leadership task was to orchestrate a sense of crisis so as to mobilize energy. One route that personnel in some authorities used from the early days was to agitate at a national policy-making level. This was easier for the high prevalence authorities, which had been early into using the media and developing high level national links. Key clinicians took advantage of their expert status to press the case: 'We are in a situation where we do have a public health crisis – in fact the greatest public health crisis that any of us in our professional lives have ever seen.' (Clinical product champion giving evidence to the House of Commons Social Services Committe 1987).

In the long term, however, such a hectic pace could not always be sustained – the HIV/AIDS issue became intractable in its turn: 'By mid-1985 we were a publishing house, a health education house as well as a treatment house, and we were very rapidly becoming exhausted.'

It proved important, also, to try to ensure that the issue was not oversold. As the pace of the epidemic seemed to slow in 1988 and 1989, so there was an increasing view that the AIDS 'crisis' was apparent rather than real (and indeed some of the local crises had been artfully constructed). Initial, and very ambitious, extrapolations of the need for beds were vulnerable to downward revision when the predicted number of patients failed to materialize, leading to doctors being accused of making 'exaggerated claims' for increased resources and seeing HIV/AIDS purely as: 'An opportunity for the development of [their] wards and for the better recognition of their specialty'.

By 1989, the momentum and energy produced by the sense of crisis were dissipating and a number of early innovators were withdrawing from the field. Some, inveterate entrepreneurs, went because of the attraction of still newer issues, such as the implementation of the White Paper, *Working for Patients*. Others were seen to be pulling back and delegating much of the work they had originally done themselves to others. Some of these were simply exhausted through overcommitment, but others had made their names and reputations in AIDS and were now moving in more exalted circles. Although most champions were clearly committed to an altruistic vision of combating the epidemic, it is inescapable that their motives for involvement were not unmixed with personal advancement. Many of those scorned by their contemporaries for their early obsession with HIV/AIDS – 'he's on his hobby horse again' – have more recently seen their hunches justified by invitations to sit on national committees as experts, international recognition and offers of prestigious new appointments. In addition, many have seen their specialties expanded and transformed by new capital and revenue money.

Concluding discussion

In Chapter 5 we considered how it was that a new and very unusual health care issue (HIV/AIDS) was 'sensed' and brought into existing public sector organizations or even used to create completely new voluntary organizations. At this very early stage of the change cycle, a small number of actors were involved, many of whom could be seen as visionaries, deviants and heretics. Few were securely placed at the centre of their organizations. Although clinicians could trade on the social prestige that they enjoyed to influence events, those clinicians drawn into the emerging HIV/AIDS field were generally working in historically marginal specialties.

In this chapter, we have considered the subsequent question of how broader forms of activity were launched in the emerging field of HIV/ AIDS. A number of mechanisms were identified whereby a broader level of concern was developed. Clearly the provision of earmarked central funds was vital in legitimating local activity, although the provision of these funds itself followed on from intensive lobbying at the centre. The sense of 'crisis', also, at least in the medium term, had energizing effects and helped erode traditional organizational boundaries. A common 'strong culture' was apparent in a number of different HIV/AIDS service settings, with the result that apparently isolated services were bound together by normative glue. Some of the most effective 'product champions' had strong coalition building skills.

At a more general level, there is a question of how innovating groups – in general – survive in the world while changing it (see Pettigrew (1985) for a discussion of the fate of innovating and value-laden organizational development groups). The legitimacy of the activity and credibility of individual practitioners, especially of advisory services, which cannot command line authority, has to be developed and maintained over time if the activity is to flourish.

Some previous research (Pettigrew 1975) has suggested that specialist groups may typically display a task orientated and politically limited perspective. Over time, such a group may move from a self-confident pioneering stage to one characterized by self-doubt:

> Only when the certainty of the original pioneering task nears completion, and uncertainties about future tasks and political sponsorship for the group become starkly evident, do groups of innovators sit down, often by then in an atmosphere of collective self doubt, and begin to try and put together a home and foreign policy.
>
> (Pettigrew 1985: 506)

At this point, such innovating groups face a dilemma between 'exclusive' and 'inclusive' approaches to the management of their boundaries with the wider system. The exclusive stance is characterized by the following features:

- little permeability of boundary;
- cultural dissimilarity;
- specific values;
- unilateral exchanges with environment;
- limited network and linkages;
- limited range of transactions with environment.

The inclusive stance, on the other hand, is characterized by:

- highly permeable boundary;
- cultural similarity;
- diffuse values;
- mutual exchanges with environment;
- well-developed network and linkages;
- broad range of transactions with environment.

The innovative group behaving the exclusive stance is offering a distinctively sharp and culturally deviant presentation of itself to the wider environment. It may well be influenced by the 'zealots', who have proved so useful in the early stages of the change process by breaking up the inertia that so often characterizes large organizations. While such a stance may be useful in maintaining a distinctive group identity, there is the risk of obtaining little influence over the rest of the system.

The alternative strategy is to behave the inclusive stance, which:

... is the behavioural expression of the aphorism that to change the world one must live with it. Here is the attempt literally to change the world by inclusion in it, to understand and where appropriate identify with local cultures and to use such cultural identification to cultivate the access and information which will reveal the pragmatic starting point or points for change.

(Pettigrew 1985: 508)

Here the dangers are those of excessive absorption and cooptation, leading to a loss of drive for change. Innovating groups may of course mix the two strategies, perhaps moving from exclusive to inclusive stances over time. The dilemma is to be different enough to create change but not so different so as to create a moral panic, or be labelled as 'folk devils'.

How can we classify the newly developed HIV/AIDS specialist services studied using this classification? Our broad view is that many more of them – despite the existence of a strong common culture, which is usually seen as a feature of an 'exclusive' stance – should be seen as adopting a broadly inclusive stance.

The network form of organization meant that the natural allies, which were scattered throughout different services, could be spotted and cultivated. Staff in AIDS services were good at moving from one service setting to another (e.g. dentistry, genitourinary medicine, prisons). They were typically adept at winning resources from the wider system for their programmes, even if this meant moving towards a more managerialized form of organization (Patton 1990), which contradicted their earlier practice. They were skilled at 'managing up', and lobbying key power centres, and many also demonstrated a flair for managing the media.

This was a relative rather than absolute inclusiveness as a number of AIDS services settings, for instance, demonstrated good links with other public sector settings (e.g. the youth service) but weaker links with, say, private sector employers. Nevertheless a number of them were working at developing links with prison and police services, which typically displayed very different value systems from those apparent in HIV/AIDS services. This relative sophistication in boundary management was an important factor in the broadening of the base from the initial visionaries and heretics.

HAROLD BRIDGES LIBRARY
S. MARTIN'S COLLEGE
LANCASTER

CHAPTER
7

Working across boundaries

Introduction

The interorganizational context

The theme of this chapter, working across boundaries, is a subject of substantial management interest and also of academic analysis. Within the private sector, there is a growing interest in the analysis of such phenomena as interorganizational networks, strategic alliances and internationalization processes (Harrigan 1988; Lyles 1990), all of which involve the crossing of organizational boundaries.

Within the public sector – and especially health and social care services – there is also increasing interest in the properties of various kinds of policy networks (Rhodes 1988), and there has been a long-running concern with problems of 'coordination' (or more realistically lack of coordination) between different public agencies (Booth 1981; Webb 1991). This presenting problem of 'lack of coordination' quickly raises much deeper questions of processes of interorganizational exchange (explored as long ago as 1961, by Levine and White) between different agencies. This is now so well-established a theme in public sector settings that the periodic calls for more coordination may sometimes be seen as no more than an exercise in symbolic politics, which need not lead to substantive action.

Why should this problem of lack of coordination be so evident in health care? Many illnesses require care and treatment from a multiplicity of settings, thus raising the question of case collaboration at operational level. Where this fails, 'revolving door' patterns of discharge and readmission may emerge. At a more strategic level, questions of agency role and responsibility, and of policy and flows of finance arise, for example, between health services, social services and voluntary organizations. Where effective collaboration does not exist at this strategic level, there may well be 'cost shunting' between these different agencies, as each tries to offload responsibilities and costs onto the others. Each of the three types of agency exhibits different models of care, financing mechanisms, decision-making processes and arrangements for corporate governance.

The long-standing 'grey areas' apparent in health and social care (e.g. the unclear division of labour between district nursing and local authority home care services; Davies et al. 1990: Chapter 8) add to the complexity. Service personnel negotiate between themselves at a local level as to which tasks rightfully belong to which agency. This is overlaid by a declared but only partially implemented policy shift (DHSS 1976) to move the overall focus of care from hospital to community care settings, which from 1976 onwards was aided by the provision of special incentives through the introduction of joint finance monies. Successfully transferring lead responsibility from health to social care was a central task in the management of the closure and reprovision of mental handicap hospitals in the late 1980s (Pettigrew et al. 1992: Chapter 7). Disappointment with the patchy effects of joint finance (Cm 849 1989) led eventually to the creation of a more explicit 'lead agency' model in which social services departments were to be seen as prime managers in the field of community care. However, this lead agency model still does not resolve the difficulties inherent in the provision of care and treatment for people who move in and out of hospital and community-based settings.

Joint working and the HIV/AIDS issue

The policy context into which the new HIV/AIDS issue emerged was thus one that ostensibly favoured interorganizational working. However, given the disjuncture noted by Webb (1991) between the rhetoric of policy and the observed behaviour of practice in this area, it is interesting that the need for 'jointness' of service provision for HIV/AIDS was apparently recognized from the beginning by practitioners (often clinicians dealing with patients) convening early *ad hoc* working groups on AIDS, as well as by policy makers.

Medical factors indicating a need for collaboration and cross-boundary working included: the number of separate medical specialties involved in caring for the many different parts of the body affected by HIV disease; the nature of HIV/AIDS as an increasingly chronic illness, suggesting the need to plan and coordinate patient care with primary care teams, paramedical and social care teams; and the lack of knowledge about this completely new illness, facilitating the development of more reciprocal relationships with patients and with voluntary organizations. Preventative measures, also, could not be rapidly and effectively addressed by standard public health and infection control techniques, but required the involvement of many other agencies in order to address behaviours that are under private rather than public control.

Nor could the issue be treated just as an illness. As Aggleton and Homans (1988) argue, the social aspects of HIV/AIDS range from the personal psychological effects of being diagnosed as HIV-positive to the many social systems, practices and processes on which it impinges. From schools to prisons, businesses to tourist boards, it is harder to identify groups and organizations that did *not* need to be involved than those that did. Furthermore, many of those personally affected by HIV/AIDS, in particular the gay community, were able to organize themselves to demand recognition of their social and emotional needs, and the opportunity to collaborate in the management of the issue, in a way which would have been unthinkable in previous epidemics.

Official circles were also supportive of an interorganizational approach to HIV/AIDS. For example, the Commons Social Services Committee report (1987) on AIDS made it quite explicit that the response to HIV should not be confined to the health service, but should go further. It recommended that: '. . . local authorities and health authorities at all levels establish joint planning procedures . . .' (recommendation 65) and that: '. . . the role of the voluntary sector needs to be recognized and coordinated with that of the statutory sector' (recommendation 92).

For all these reasons, working across organizational boundaries has been an important theme in the response to HIV/AIDS. It is of interest because we are here moving beyond established and routinized coordination patterns to consider patterns of interorganizational change (Webb 1991). In the rest of this chapter, we briefly review some literature and then use our empirical data to examine the factors that affected cross-boundary working in HIV/AIDS and consider to what extent they may illuminate and extend our knowledge of collaborative working in general.

Interorganizational conflict and cooperation

How should we attempt to analyse processes of interorganizational cooperation and conflict within public sector settings? Webb (1991) starts his own analysis by outlining three alternative explanatory frameworks: (1) imperative or mandated coordination; (2) the rational altruistic model; and (3) the bargaining exchange model of bureaucratic politics. He does not suggest that these are mutually exclusive, or that they account for all the observed variance in the organizational processes, but that they represent the 'ebb and flow of academic debate' and can be seen as both partially explaining and affecting practice. Certainly it is possible to identify examples of each of these patterns of collaboration within the development of services for HIV/AIDS.

Imperative or mandated coordination

Imperative or mandated coordination involves intervention through the authority or power of the higher tiers of the state to require lower tier organizations to coordinate their activities, or at least to be seen to be so doing. This pattern was evident in the field of joint planning in the 1970s. However, such joint committees were widely seen as of marginal signifi-cance (Booth 1981), and Webb (1991) argues that there is a history of failure to achieve coordination through such means in novel situations, as they may go against the grain of pre-existing cultures and practices and across the boundaries of autonomous professions. Nevertheless, in prag-matic terms, the imposition of such a framework may sometimes be effec-tive in compelling acknowledgement of, and some response, however limited, to a particular issue. As we discuss later, with HIV/AIDS, action had emerged through organic, bottom-up processes in only a few health au-thorities prior to the Department of Health circular requiring the setting up of a committee structure in 1986, until then the rest had largely failed to react, despite the clear relevance of aspects of the issue to all of them.

Rational altruism

Another pattern identified by Webb is that of rational altruism. This model combines elements of the rational synoptic approach to planning and notions of organizational altruism (Challis et al. 1988). Webb sees it as exemplified by the attempts at long-range strategic planning in the 1960s and 1970s. The model requires actors to maintain a long-term and system-wide view-point and for all parties to accept at least some overarching goals and objectives. It also assumes that actors are willing to set aside sectional goals in favour of the wider good.

Although the rhetoric is appealing, it often seems difficult to maintain such a purposive approach in reality, particularly at an organizational level. However, for small groups with a mission, this would seem to be a model with some explanatory power and certainly some of those involved in developing service for HIV/AIDS would fit this description.

Bargaining and exchange

As Webb points out, the reality of self-interest (often operating alongside more altruistic motivations) cannot be ignored, and the third model –

bargaining and exchange – assumes that, in real life, organizations are dominated by micropolitical processes. Departments compete against each other for funds and for political attention; professions compete with each other for turf. As such, this perspective has much face validity. However, Webb (1991) notes that it has been critiqued for its tendency to reductionism, a narrow view of the motivational basis of action, while others have attacked an alleged overconcentration on the minutiae of exchange, rather than broad structural factors.

Sometimes such organizational exchange has been seen within the context of unequal power relationships, creating power on the one side and dependency on the other (Blau 1964; Rhodes 1988). There may here be relations of domination, but not of genuine cooperation. This helps embed the analysis of a particular bargaining relation within a wider consideration of the unequal distribution of power. This more structural perspective can be helpful. Clearly, for example, consultant clinicians can be seen as possessing substantial power and status, which may facilitate their attempts to cross conventional organizational boundaries. However, like Webb, we would question the validity of a wholly determinist perspective: what is striking is how different the outcomes of attempts to secure joint working are, rather than how similar. One locality reports moves towards joint strategies, while another reports very little progress indeed. Nor is it easy to apply a simple power-dependence model to concrete interorganizational exchanges. Indeed, a frequent criticism of the joint finance programme was that although the NHS provided the resources, local government controlled the spend. Processes then seem to retain an emergent character that is not captured by these mechanistic models.

Although the bureaucratic politics model identified by Webb seems to contain some descriptive validity, it may require further reshaping. There is perhaps an increasing awareness of the importance of other micro-organizational factors – besides bargaining processes – in shaping the degree of joint working. The importance of 'reticulists' or boundary spanners has long been apparent (Friend et al. 1974; confirmed in Pettigrew et al. 1992). There is an increasing interest in the role of cross-organizational networks and Rhodes (1988) identifies a typology of different networks, although in our opinion the ideological basis of these networks does not appear to have been well explored. For instance, where people hold similar beliefs, attitudes and values, this may be a far better predictor of cooperation than their individual allegiance to any particular organization or even professional group, as illustrated by Lofland's (1971) 'horizontal cliques', which formed across departments in pursuit of a particular valued goal.

Webb's own analysis concludes by emphasizing the role of trust (Webb 1991) in determining outcomes of joint working. He sees trust as pivotal to collaboration, generating the courage required to make initial approaches to others perceived as operating in different modes, and needing to be reinforced as joint ventures expand and involve greater degrees of risk. Trust is, of course, situated in attitudes, beliefs and values, providing a bridge across the uncertainties inherent in situations and relationships. March and Olsen (1976) see it as crucial to operating under conditions of ambiguity. In the absence of concrete evidence, organizational participants vary in their perceptions according to whether or not they trust the sources of such information as is available to them, and their view of reality is formed through these relationships.

This suggests that in reviewing the data collected on the development of cross-boundary working in relation to HIV/AIDS, we also need to consider some more subjective or perceptual influences on patterns of joint working, for example, ideology, organizational culture, knowledge base and shared experience, as the key to whether trust developed or not may lie in large measure in the specific history and experience of the small groups set up to process the issue.

Thus the HIV/AIDS issue can be seen as having created a complex organizational field moulded as much by informal processes involving relationships, beliefs and perceptions, as by formal structures, resources and policies. Nowhere is this more marked than in the complicated inter- and intraorganizational networks involved in the development of cross-boundary working. In the following sections we explore in greater detail the facilitating and inhibiting effects of some of these factors on the development of services.

Organizational boundaries and HIV/AIDS services

The first and most basic point to make is that HIV/AIDS services are indeed characterized by a multiplicity of agency and service boundaries. The effective crossing of these boundaries is a critical management task and at the very least much lip service has been paid to securing joint working within HIV/AIDS services. Some small early groups achieved good collaborative working patterns, but many of those attempting to initiate a more structured joint approach have found profound obstacles and barriers to cooperation. No 'lead agency' model has emerged in HIV/AIDS services, unlike (say) mental handicap services, to simplify these problems of coordination. We here illustrate the general problem by focusing on four characteristic scenarios that have emerged in a number of localities.

First, the difficulties of cross-service cooperation can be particularly acute in localities where a plethora of small, ideologically driven, specialist teams have grown up organically in response to funding opportunities. Even where interteam cooperation is indicated, ideological conflict and competition for clients may make it difficult to cross such team boundaries. (See Cranfield et al. (1992), for a discussion of this problem in drugs services on one case study locality, where some services operated according to an abstinence model and others on a harm reduction basis.)

A second problem is that catchment areas for patients often cross a number of health authority, local authority and voluntary organization boundaries. Much time may be spent negotiating separately with each different organization, and attempts to secure short cuts may be illusory. This interorganizational network, therefore, can be highly complex, especially in the case of teaching hospitals and large voluntary organizations:

> [At the moment it is] nightmarish. We have spent all of every week . . . turning up to working parties with [different] local authorities arguing our case, and something is deferred until the following week and if you can't make it you come back next time and it has all been rewritten . . . As we have a . . . [regional health grant] we ought to cover the whole of the region . . . [but] we are at the wrong end geographically.
>
> (manager of a voluntary sector organization)

A third issue relates to the effects of different flows of finance on interorganizational behaviour. While these financial issues tend to become a particular concern for senior management rather than front line practitioners, the hierarchy may nevertheless try to restrain 'overcooperative' behaviour at case level if it is likely to place the organization at a severe financial disadvantage. While some health authorities were allocated some special central funding for HIV/AIDS services as early as 1985, it was only in 1988 that local authorities were offered a support grant to cover 70 per cent of their expenditure on the issue. Even then, they were to remain responsible for picking up the remaining 30 per cent of their expenditure.

A fourth issue was particularly important for some health education teams. The interorganizational network and the number of potential stakeholders that they faced was so diffuse and vast that somehow choices had to be made in deciding which links were of priority importance. So some linkages in the diffuse interorganizational network may become defined as of more importance than others. But how is this to be done? Are large private sector employers more or less important than prisons? Should attention be concentrated on the education service or on youth clubs?

Mandated coordination

Reviewing the material collected in the case study localities, our general view is that the formal joint planning machinery has had, on the whole, only modest impact. This is a disappointing but unsurprising finding, reflecting what we already know about the impact of mandated coordination in other fields.

As early as 1986, the DHSS issued a Circular directing 'standing action groups' on AIDS to be constituted formally in every health authority: '... accountable to the health authority through a nominated community physician, to be responsible for coordinating relevant local services and spearheading prevention.' This signalled a shift towards an overall coordinating function being undertaken by public health and away from the early clinical product champions. It entailed a wider and more structural view being taken of boundary management, removing the focus from key personalities and small groups and creating more formal structures where each agency had a right to representation. Sometimes this machinery was complemented with joint planning bodies, but usually without control over significant levels of resource. Public health physicians often had prior experience of joint working and some were enthusiastic in their attempts to apply this model in the field of HIV/AIDS.

However, in the judgement of the researchers, there was only a minority of localities studied where such mandated joint bodies could be seen as effective and as influential. In one of these, the Department of Health circular was used by the Director of Public Health to engineer a shift from an early infection control focus to wider aspects of prevention and care. A new committee was set up with wide representation from general management, the health promotion department and the community drugs team, and also including the voluntary sector and the local authority. The voluntary sector representatives here were influential members of the joint steering group, partly because the City Council was under left-wing Labour control, with close working relationships with SMOs.

Another locality had made deliberate moves towards more substantive power-sharing on their joint committee, using such devices as rotation of the role of chair. Here important changes in behaviour towards 'jointness' could be discerned:

> I think what has happened is that people have been prepared to give up power and a few things that normally get in the way of good liaison and joint planning and so on, which has been very helpful ... So we've managed to go forward together, and I think, as long as the personalities don't change ... I think that will serve us well for a long time.
>
> (social services respondent)

These examples were, however, in the minority. In most localities, such joint planning bodies were often seen as ineffective or as 'rubber stamps':

> It's far too big to do any planning at all. It's got to involve five health districts, ten different voluntary organizations, which are all crucial, the local authority, and seven different departments of the local authority, there is absolutely no way that group can plan. It also has very little influence on the organizations that are represented there,

it seems to me to only serve the function of a limited information exchange and meeting the requirements that most of us have that we ought to be trying to work together.

(social services respondent)

Some such groups rapidly declined as key power figures exited, with maybe one or two meetings a year and large numbers of non-attenders:

It [the Joint Care Planning Team] had about sixty people, with the voluntary sector on it, and all the medics and all the council and everybody else . . . You had lots of people at managerial level who never communicated anything at that meeting to anybody else . . . so it seemed to be a bit of a fossil, a bit of a dinosaur, and gradually you found people drifting off and not bothering to turn up . . . A lot of very important people, medics and what have you, stopped going and now it's down to about twenty people.

(health service respondent)

Where a large body of this sort existed it was inevitably too large and disparate for effective decision making. As a consequence, a small 'core' group frequently emerged, often health dominated, and from which social services and voluntary sector representatives were sometimes excluded.

In an example from one inner London locality, there was a slow start in moving towards formal joint planning. The issue became increasingly important in 1988 and 1989, however, as more non-NHS resources came on stream. A tripartite body (health, social services and voluntary sector) was therefore set up in October 1989 with an ambitious brief, but where each constituent body firmly retained its own identity:

- To identify services at the interface of all constituent bodies.
- To identify gaps in those services.
- To take such action as is necessary to bring these to the attention of the appropriate planning groups for AIDS in each constituent body, via the Joint Consultative Committee.
- To monitor and evaluate progress in achieving the action identified.
- To coordinate proposals for joint finance in relation to AIDS services in liaison with the appropriate planning groups for AIDS in each constituent body.
- To act as an information exchange between constituent bodies.

A number of important weaknesses, which were symptomatic of the body's peripheral status, soon became evident: meetings were infrequent; there was rapid turnover, including of the Chair; there was little administrative support and little executive authority or access to money: 'As an information exchange, it has been useful. In terms of actually getting down to any joint planning, we have not really got to grips with that yet' (social services representative).

Informal organizational processes

On the whole, in the localities studied, formal attempts to engineer joint working within HIV/AIDS services from the centre generally had very limited success, although a minority of more positive counterexamples could be cited. Informal aspects of organizational life, however, were seen as potentially more important in shaping the extent of joint working. These factors can be seen as informal, perceptual or subjective, in contrast to the formal structures outlined above. We consider both facilitating informal factors (e.g. crisis mentality) and inhibiting ones (e.g. differing knowledge bases) in turn.

Facilitating factors

A receptive context
In some localities, there seemed to be a 'receptive context' (Pettigrew et al. 1992) for the development of interagency working. Some localities had already developed a strong track record in working across sectoral boundaries. Local political regimes and the strength and weakness of social movements locally were also important contextual factors.

In terms of people to provide leadership for the new issue, there might be a pre-existing team (in one case a research team that had formed around hepatitis B was able to move quickly on to HIV/AIDS). A strong public health department might quickly go on to develop an interest in the policy side of the epidemic. A key factor was the potential availability of a clinical product champion, and it was not always easy to predict in advance who this was likely to be.

Boundary spanners
'Boundary spanners' existed in a number of localities, particularly between the statutory and voluntary sectors. We did not find the total separation between public sector bureaucracies and SMOs that we had perhaps expected initially. Some staff moved from voluntary organizations into posts in the HIV labour market, emerging in the NHS. On the other side, some NHS or social services staff were also actively involved in advising or indeed running voluntary organizations in their spare time. In some localities, it was possible to identify a small core group of staff, crossing conventional agency divides, with strong formal and informal links.

A shared ideology
We considered the variety of belief systems apparent in the field of HIV/AIDS in Chapter 4. Here we note the existence of strong interorganizational networks based on belief in radical ideologies, often derived from social movements. There was an almost cell-like structure evident in some

localities, with cells operating within each agency, but with strong interpersonal and informal linkages. Important shared values included an emphasis on 'empowerment' of the user, questioning of the traditional expertise of doctors and belief in the virtue of 'alternative' therapies. Services should be seen to be non-discriminatory and non-stigmatizing. Networks were to be preferred to hierarchies, although informal power figures sometimes emerged to conduct the network.

Of course, people play many roles and profess many beliefs. What is unusual about the belief systems apparent in HIV/AIDS is the degree of conviction with which they were held. They became master beliefs and master roles which over-rode other considerations. Loyalty to the HIV network could be more important than loyalty to one's discipline or work organization.

For example, one multiagency group operating in the field of AIDS education could be seen initially as exceptionally energetic, close knit, yet also fluid and non-hierarchical. Early on in its life history, it could be seen as a good example of an energetic, ideologized, network. However, strong routinization and lifecycle effects set in, and the level of energy in the network dropped:

> A factor which contributed to [the group's] early success was the ability to combine both formal and informal ways of working and to use them to their best advantage. Later, as the informal aspects of the group reached their natural life span and the Group shrank both in size and in terms of the time, energy and commitment people were able to provide, the formal aspects of the group were not sufficient to maintain cohesion and momentum.
>
> (Kleiman 1989)

Espoused ideology of joint working
Another important feature of HIV/AIDS services has been the strength of the espoused ideology of joint working. Existing joint care planning models have been imprinted in the new field of HIV/AIDS, particularly where community medicine has played a role in service planning. In part this is also because there has been strong pressure to contain the number of acute beds and to deliver community-based forms of care. An active and assertive voluntary sector has emerged as a major deliverer of such services, reinforcing the rhetoric of joint working from another quarter. AIDS Control Act returns, for instance, wax lyrically about the progress that the locality has achieved in joint working. This discourse may to some degree be rhetorical, but the rhetoric is all pervasive, and may eventually have shaped behaviour and even attitudes.

This ideology is also reflected in some of the key service settings (e.g. genitourinary medicine clinics, drug dependency units, acute wards), where the preferred form of organization is usually the 'multidisciplinary team'.

Of course, some players in the team have more power than the others (e.g. the consultant). Nevertheless, such groupings may well include not only doctors and nurses but also social workers, psychologists, health educators and volunteers, and this pluralism has shaped the model of care observable in these settings which is often far wider than the traditional concerns of biomedicine.

Clinical product champions as diplomats

We have already highlighted the role of early clinical product champions in pushing for service development in the field of HIV/AIDS. A key part of this innovatory activity – essentially the diplomatic component of the product champion role – lay in the effective crossing of conventional organizational boundaries.

An important task undertaken by the early product champions was the formation of *ad hoc* committees, essentially local and voluntary coalitions of interest. They made explicit efforts to involve people and organizations, not only outside their own specialties, but outside the health service altogether. For example, in one of our case study localities, a committee that met in the genitourinary medicine department in 1983 had membership drawn from the local authority environmental health department, the education department, community medicine, several different hospital specialties, the local voluntary phone line, and people with HIV infection themselves.

The lending of status: the umbrella of patronage

However, not all doctors have equal status, and this has been important in the field of HIV/AIDS, which has frequently had most impact on the traditionally less powerful specialties. While medicine is a high-status, professionalized occupation in its own right, it traditionally carries within it a ranking system that confers extra prestige and hence autonomy on some of its members. The status hierarchy is in part explicit (i.e. there are different grades of doctors, from house officers to consultants); but it is in part implicit, though clearly understood by members of the profession, and is based on the different specialties or 'segments' (Bucher and Strauss 1961) to which individual doctors become affiliated in the course of their careers.

In effect each segment contains a separate organizational identity and its members become closer to one another than they are to doctors in other specialties (Friedson 1970). Bucher and Stelling (1977) argue that major pressures for conflict may arise between segments, in contrast to other and more functionalist views of professions, which stress their cohesiveness and collegiality.

Status, or the lack of it, may affect the dynamics of collaborative working. Early clinical product champions were at least perceived as high status outside the walls of the hospital, if not originally internally. However, if they possessed organizational and diplomatic skills, they might also be able to use the resources and profile increasingly associated with the HIV/ AIDS issue to increase the prestige of their specialty and to form a new professional 'segment' with other consultant colleagues. Such consultant to consultant links were important in increasing the legitimacy of the HIV/ AIDS issue in hospital settings.

These early clinical product champions also used their high status to perform an important patronage role. Why did the new generation of HIV/ AIDS specialist workers in the late 1980s, the 'coordinators' and 'liaison officers' make such an impact, when, as noted in Chapter 6, they occupied relatively lowly positions within their organizational hierarchies and had little access to extra resources? Their posts were, of course, designed to be 'reticulist' in nature (Friend et al. 1974) and their job titles indicated the expectation that they would act as boundary spanners, although the extent to which they were in practice able to discharge these lateral functions depended on the micropolitics of the organization. However, a major factor in the high profile they achieved was undoubtedly the patronage of these posts by the product champions, who had often been personally involved in their appointments.

The way in which key medical professionals were sometimes able to 'lend' status to others without medical qualifications is interesting, since although this process has been described in terms of patronage *within* the medical profession (Hall 1949; Friedson 1970), there has been little discussion of the possibility of this being effective across wider boundaries. However, the proposition that powerful sponsorhip was an important factor in the influence wielded by early HIV specialist boundary spanners, is further evidenced by current circumstances. As resources in more localities have come on-stream thanks to central funding, many newly recruited HIV specialists are working in localities where there is no supportive power figure. Such workers, with little status of their own, are finding that they are much less influential at management level, and many are becoming progressively disenchanted with their inability to affect service development.

Crisis mentality
The development of a perception of crisis around HIV/AIDS also favoured cooperation, and there was an apparent period of unity in which differences between groups were transcended, reaching its peak during the time of the highly publicized government health education campaign in January 1987. Almost as dominant as the metaphor of AIDS as a 'plague' has been the use of the terminology of war (Sontag 1988), in particular, of an unwanted but just war which must be fought to ensure survival. Thus we have such titles as *The Challenge of AIDS for the Community* (BMA/RCN Conference, Cardiff, 1990); *Coping with Change in the NHS: A Frontline*

District's Response to AIDS (Ferlie and Pettigrew 1990) and *The Welsh AIDS Campaign*; while accounts of the epidemic are peppered with references to *mobilizing forces* and *championing the cause*, to say nothing of *strategies*, *tactics* and *targets*. This feeling of unifying mission favoured cooperation – at least during the short crisis phase – and was thus particularly experienced by those involved in the issue in early 1987, as one respondent recalled: 'I remember that everyone worked incredibly hard ... we had an enormous mixture of people ... there was a sense of working together and responding in a crisis, you know, the kind of thing that we English people do rather well.' There is here perhaps an echo of the folk lore that now surrounds the British response to the blitz in the Second World War.

Inhibiting factors

Having considered some of the informal organizational factors that facilitated joint working in the field of HIV/AIDS services, we now consider some inhibitors.

A non-receptive context

Just as some localities inherited a positive legacy from the past, in others the past played a more negative role. There seemed no simple model to explain the tenor of interorganizational relationships (e.g. a resource dependency model), but rather the pattern varied subtly from one locality to another.

Power struggles between individuals, groups of individuals, and sometimes (seemingly) whole organizations, may display a history that stretches back many years, quite possibly from long before HIV emerged as an issue. Many clinicians in particular may spend their entire careers in one locality, so that interpersonal disputes are unlikely to be resolved by one party moving on but may continue for years. Such deep-seated patterns could prove difficult to change and soon imprinted themselves on the 'new' HIV/AIDS issue. This could be the case with intergroup and interorganizational conflict as well as interpersonal conflict. In some cases, relations between (say) the health service and local authorities were generally seen as poor, and it was difficult for HIV/AIDS to escape from this overall constraint. In other cases, established institutions (e.g. some drug dependency units) can be seen as having a long history of difficulty in managing service change, and these organizational pathologies were carried forward in their response to HIV/AIDS.

The characteristics of key roles

The key point here is that some of the roles that have emerged as central to the process of service development in HIV/AIDS (e.g. clinical product champion, 'bureaucratic insurgent') may produce more of a competitive than a cooperative orientation. It will be interesting to see whether the introduction of quasi markets in health care will reinforce these tendencies towards competitive behaviour.

Frequently, the early clinical product champions – while embracing the concept of multidisciplinary working – also preferred to build up services within their own departments. By so doing, and while acknowledging the skills of others, they were still able to retain overall responsibility for patient care.

In consequence, specialist units began to provide an increasingly comprehensive package of services, covering inpatient, outpatient, 'drop in', respite and terminal care facilities, with testing, counselling, and various therapeutic activities all under one roof. This in fact can be seen as the antithesis of a fully cooperative model, which would seek to coordinate care through a number of specialist agencies. It is, however, true that such specialist units tended to be highly acceptable to people with HIV, as long as they were within easy reach.

This kind of 'empire building' – albeit of a kind acceptable to users – may be an important characteristic of professionalism (Wilensky 1964). It may even be true of entrepreneurial activity more generally, as research has shown that individual change agents frequently expect to achieve their ends through familiar means, and within their own span of control (Welsh and White 1981).

What is likely to be the impact on these specialist units of the recent NHS reorganization based on the principles of an internal market (Cm 555, 1989) and of gradual moves towards contracting for HIV/AIDS services? If, as has been argued (Stockford 1992), the essential purposes of the new purchasing function include taking an strategic overview of services and also shifting services from secondary into primary care, then the new arrangements should serve to enhance moves towards community-based care. The danger is that increased provider competition may encourage existing specialist acute units to attract more funding by providing an even more comprehensive service and engaging in marketing activity (we now see the emergence of sophisticated promotional material from some units specializing in HIV/AIDS services who are engaged in a 'customer care' offensive).

Old-style district committees, on the other hand, are turning into purchasing advisory groups, which can make recommendations but frequently do not take an active part in the process of contracting. Furthermore, the multidisciplinary element of their original membership may become attenuated if purchasing is seen as purely a health services function. Current trends in organization and management therefore may erode even the degree of joint working that has been achieved.

Different knowledge bases

We here refer to the reluctance of one group of experts to acknowledge the validity and usefulness of the expertise of another, and the barriers to communication and understanding that may result from the existence of different bases of expert knowledge in the same field of care and treatment. We also refer to the different forms of knowledge that are characteristic of expert and non-expert groups, and the extent to which such expert knowledge is seen as authoritative or as contestable by the lay audience.

Becher (1989) indeed uses the language of 'academic tribes and territories' in his characterization of how groups of academics often build disciplines with distinctive identities and cultures. Not only does the content of knowledge vary from one discipline to another, but at a more fundamental level even the type of knowledge accredited as authoritative (e.g. hard/soft; inductive/deductive).

These reflections on the sociology of knowledge may also be valid in relation to other knowledge-based forms of work such as the medical profession. As Bucher and Strauss (1961) argue, it is part of the nature of professionalism for the expertise of those from other disciplines, or even within disciplines, to be treated with suspicion. Pettigrew (1973), in his research on the emergence of specialist groups around the new discipline of computer programming, noted that this tends to be particularly evident when, as with HIV/AIDS, professional norms have yet to be established. In such situations there may be resistance to adapting working practices to include and involve other groups.

In HIV/AIDS, the potential for conflict around the most authoritative form of knowledge may be even greater as some radical SMOs have stressed the lived experience as the most legitimate form of knowledge, rejecting the claims to authority of the expert discourse. Stacey (1988) outlines the wide plurality of healing systems that now exist, in addition to the conventional model of biomedicine. Alternative healing systems were indeed influential in some quarters affected by the HIV/AIDS epidemic.

For example, a multidisciplinary AIDS group might contain medical and surgical representatives (perhaps working with a traditional biomedical model), a public health doctor (working with more of a community- and population-based model), a health education officer (working with a social and an educational model) and voluntary sector representatives (working to an experiential model).

Developing norms of care around HIV/AIDS are based on a much broader definition of collaboration, emphasizing a real sharing of responsibility for decision making amongst all those involved, including non-professionals such as the person with HIV and his/her carers, and the validity of different views of what was, or was not appropriate treatment. However

committed to the principle of patient choice, some medical experts have
found the logical outcomes of such a policy hard to handle. They found
themselves having work alongside practitioners of alternative therapies
they perceived to be of marginal usefulness, if not actually worthless, but
which were valued by patients. Or, as in the following quote, they found
themselves having to make detailed technical explanations to justify their
selected treatments:

> I find it difficult that I have to take every single patient through a sort
> of immunology, virology course in order to persuade them. All right,
> I talk to the patients about it and they always have the choice. But
> I do feel that they should trust me if I say to them, 'Look your
> T4 cell count is this, and there are good indications that at this level
> you should start taking AZT in a low dose, and you shouldn't have
> any problems.' If they are going to trust me to look after them when
> they are ill, then they should trust me to look after them in those
> decisions.
>
> (consultant physician)

Differences did not just concern treatment and care, opinions about
prevention and methods of achieving it also varied between disciplines.
While counsellors might see preserving confidentiality of prime importance
in ensuring that people come forward for testing and advice about prevention, surgeons have argued that they need information about people's HIV
status to protect themselves (Sim and Dudley 1988). Epidemiologists lobbied strongly for anonymous testing of blood samples from pregnant women
as an aid to estimating the prevalence of HIV in the general population,
other professionals profoundly disagreed with the concept of collecting
information without utilizing it to help individuals and refused to cooperate. Provision of injecting equipment and condoms to drug users were
obvious ways of preventing spread of infection to some, and yet were
completely unacceptable to a number of those running traditional drugs
services based on abstinence.

One professional grouping would sometimes display negative stereotypes
about the competence of other professional groupings who operated outside their own setting. For example, some doctors in acute units were
reluctant to refer to district nursing:

> The hospital consultants had no concept of what district nurses could
> do, they thought they were bathing ladies, they really had no idea
> that they are some of our most highly trained nurses, and that nearly
> all of them had been ward sisters.
>
> (nurse manager)

The same stereotyping was sometimes evident in relation to consultants'
perception of the role of GPs:

There is a conflict between community care and specialist care . . . you cannot expect people to learn how to look after AIDS until it is a bit more mature and we have got used to it a bit. So I think in long-term planning, yes I can see it in ten to fifteen years time, it will be possible to look after patients in the community, but, now, people do not know how to do it. GPs can't do it, and a lot of hospital physicians can't do it, and I think that to pretend that they can is wrong.

(consultant physician)

Different organizational forms, cultures and practices
The NHS, social care agencies and voluntary organizations operating in the field of HIV/AIDS, can all be seen as exhibiting distinctive organizational forms, cultures and working practices.

For instance, the NHS has been traditionally dominated by the powerful medical profession, albeit with a rising challenge from general management. Consumer views have usually been seen as excluded (Alford 1975). The medical profession has enjoyed substantial autonomy at the level of practice, although managers would act to ensure that financial control was maintained across the whole organization. Doctors are organized in a professional association (the British Medical Association – BMA), which in its organizational form can best be described as a professionalized bureaucracy. Non-executive directors on health authorities are appointed and not elected. There is upwards accountability to government ministers, who set the overall national policy framework, and finance is allocated nationally.

Social care agencies exhibit a weaker professional base (social work), and a stronger managerial line hierarchy. Notions of professional autonomy are weaker than in medicine. Social workers are organized in trade unions (NALGO, now UNISON) and are accountable to the local social services committee. Councillors are elected, usually on a party basis, and may be involved in the detail of policy in a way that would be considered unusual in health care. On the other hand, they may be more open to community groupings than non-executive directors in the NHS who have been often been selected for their personal expertise and track record of achievement rather than links with local community groups.

Voluntary organizations exhibit a very different organizational form, based at least in their very early stages on altruism and charisma. Bureaucratic modes of control are seen as less legitimate, and it is much more difficult to control or even 'manage' volunteers than a paid workforce. Control strategies tend to be more normative in character. Of course, initially fluid voluntary organizations may become routinized and formalized over time.

These very general differences in organizational form may be paralleled by more concrete variations in working practice. One complaint, for instance, frequently aimed by doctors at social workers is that they may not respond sufficiently quickly to requests for help in an emergency (Bennett 1989), whereas social workers may criticize doctors for failing to appreciate the need for lengthy case conferences. Workers from statutory organizations will frequently hold meetings during the working day, while workers from non-statutory sectors may only be able to attend outside normal working hours.

Personnel may experience considerable culture shock in moving from one organizational culture to another. For instance, workers recruited from SMOs into the NHS suddenly found themselves in a much more hierarchical and rule-bound organization:

> There are all kinds of bureaucratic ways of doing things that drive me completely berserk. Such as when you want to get an order for condoms, instead of ringing up the suppliers and saying 'Put them on the next train and invoice me', you have to raise an order from supplies. They then come back six weeks later and say 'you're ordering more than the family planning clinics, why is this . . . ?
>
> (health service respondent)

Experiential boundaries

In some ways, these may be the most important of all barriers to collaborative working, partly because they frequently go unrecognized or at least unarticulated. Patients experience things differently from their carers, clinicians' understanding of service needs may be qualitatively different from those of managers, workers in community services may see needs for care that would never be considered by those working in the acute sector.

The culture that has developed around HIV services has emphasized user involvement, with the aim of achieving individually tailored services and collaboration between doctors and patients on treatment regimes. It may therefore seem somewhat perverse to be suggesting that there may still be a problem in creating shared understandings between those involved. Paradoxically, though, the degree of collaboration that has been achieved may act as an invisible barrier to greater awareness by creating a degree of complacency.

Concluding discussion

Our first conclusion is that processes of joint working and of interorganizational exchange are indeed a major theme in HIV/AIDS services both for their management and analysis. Such services pose the problems of joint working in almost a classic form: a multiplicity of different agencies, settings and professional groupings are all involved in the delivery of service.

Moreover, it seems unlikely that this interorganizational complexity can be much reduced. A 'lead agency' model is difficult to apply in HIV/AIDS services, where patients may unpredictably move between hospital and community care. While the emergence of specialist acute units delivering a range of different services would provide a lead setting, this development is likely to be discouraged by purchasers seeking to develop cheaper and more local community-based alternatives.

Our second conclusion is that there were generally only modest returns secured from those formal structures set up on the basis of cooperation mandated from the top. This confirms what has been found from other studies of joint planning machinery (Webb 1991). Nevertheless, it is concerning that the world of policy making has not engaged with available research evidence. If public services do not generate more of a capacity for organizational learning, then badly designed wheels will keep on being reinvented.

Third, we found that a high degree of informal cooperation has been achieved, particularly at the level of the service setting rather than strategic management. The 'multidisciplinary team' was a characteristic mode of organization in many genitourinary clinics, drugs services and indeed hospital wards.

This finding directs us to the importance of the informal organization as a determinant of patterns of joint working. It also confirms the results of other groups. For instance, the evaluation by Kleiman (1989: 57) of a group involved in HIV/AIDS education concluded that the group evaluated had been operating in formal organizational systems that appeared, on the whole, to be resistant to the concept of multiagency and multidisciplinary approaches to work. Even where there was support in theory, it proved extremely difficult to translate that theory into practice. That is not to say that joint working did not occur. It did, and frequently. The important point was that it occurred usually in spite of, and not because of, formal decision-making systems.

A number of informal organizational factors were discussed as shapers of processes of joint working. We highlighted the importance of the ideologically informed network. In any future work, we would want to concentrate on studying the processes and outcomes of small joint groups operating in this field. While we feel that the level of trust within these groups is indeed important (Webb 1991), we need to understand more about which contexts produce high levels of trust. Good (1988), for instance, suggests that cooperation is more likely on any one occasion or issue where interaction is a long-term prospect or necessity, where large initial stakes are avoided and where communication exists over a wide range of other issues. Presumably the issue of group power also arises as actors are unlikely to invest time in a joint group, which – however trustworthy – is unable to implement its proposals. Such groups are likely to be a continuing feature of HIV/AIDS services and are worthy of further analysis.

There is also the broader question of the development of trust where, of necessity, joint working needs legitimation and implementation at a corporate level. Will it always depend on small cabals of those with close relationships and mutual interests presenting *fait accompli* to the larger group; or are there any mechanisms which can work with a larger, more representative, constituency and not leave anyone feeling their concerns have not been considered?

HIV/AIDS, adaptation and learning

Introduction

Not only is HIV/AIDS a new illness caused by a previously unknown virus, but it is also a new health care issue, requiring the development of innovative services, the radical reappraisal of some methods of service delivery and traditional attitudes and the devising of approaches to forward planning under conditions of great uncertainty. The response to HIV/AIDS, therefore, may be seen as a good example of whether individuals, groups and indeed organizations as a whole can adapt to new circumstances under conditions of crisis, uncertainty and continuing change or even, in a more abstract sense, use the experience to learn how to respond to change.

For many years there has been considerable interest in the processes by which those in organizations may collectively adapt to environmental pressures and learn new ways of behaving in response to a changing environment. Writers on organizational change sometimes refer to adaptation as if it is almost synonymous with learning. For instance, de Geus (1988) poses the question 'How does a company learn and adapt?' and then goes on to ask 'Why are some companies better able to adapt?' However, there are problems with using the two terms interchangeably. An adaptive response to a particular stimulus may be different every time the stimulus is applied, whereas a learned response, (and here we follow Bass and Vaughan's (1966) parsimonious definition of learning as a relatively stable change in behaviour occurring as a result of experience), implies an acquired reaction which is linked to, and results from, a particular stimulus.

Thus organizational learning can be seen as a change in the collective behaviour of all or some of those within an organization in response to a particular situation. However, this defines learning as essentially a reactive process. Another, rather newer, focus of interest in the literature on processes of organizational adaptation and learning is the concept of 'the learning organization'. Under its original title of 'the learning company', Pedler et al. (1988) promote the concept as almost a different organizational form, defining it as: '. . . an organization which facilitates the learning of all its members *and* [their emphasis] continuously transforms itself'. This takes the notion of collective learning several steps forward, suggesting that under certain conditions an organizational environment may be created in which processes of learning and change are actively and consciously promoted.

Much recent work has moved learning theory away from an emphasis on conditioning and motivation. New work now stresses 'experiential learning', 'self and group development' and 'collective organizational learning', which results from flatter organizational structures (see Jones and Hendry's useful (1992) review of the field). However, their focus is more on programmatic interventions (how can management create a learning organization?), whereas the learning opportunities in the field of HIV/AIDS are much more bottom-up, emergent and outwith formal management control.

This seems to suggest three different processes by which organizations may respond to new circumstances. Two are reactive – organizational adaptation and organizational learning – and the third – the development of the learning organization – is a proactive process. Each has its own particular niche in the literature on organizational change, though there is clearly some degree of overlap and the concepts are sometimes used interchangeably. Hedberg (1981) endorses this view, though using the terms defensive and offensive adjustment rather than reactive and proactive learning.

However, there is something that may serve to both link and separate these concepts in a way that is helpful to those studying processes of organizational change, the influence of time. It may be argued that the essence of each of these change processes, adaptation and reactive and proactive organizational learning, is that they represent a sequence of events. Using this approach, adaptation represents the initial, more or less unconsidered, response to a new stimulus (the classic 'knee-jerk' reaction). Reactive learning comes next, with one of possibly a number of different adaptive responses becoming a learned way of behaving in a particular situation. Finally, if the stimulus is sufficiently persistent and perceived as important to the organization, conscious steps may be taken to promote a general organizational response in a particular direction.

In this chapter, then, we argue that it may be helpful, when considering organizational change, to think of processes of organizational adaptation and reactive and proactive learning, as qualitatively different, and often temporally separate. In support of this, we explore the links and discontinuities between these processes by considering evidence from our empirical work on the development of services for HIV/AIDS. Initially we consider the nature of the work context and argue that the NHS should in general be seen as a forgetting rather than a learning organization. We then discuss to what extent the early reaction to news of the epidemic in our authorities illustrates generic processes of adaptation to a sudden and unexpected change in the organizational environment. In the following section, we look at how people and groups learned to respond in particular ways to the new situation. Following that, we consider whether a more fundamental and proactive learning process is now beginning to take place as a result of the recognition that issues raised by developing services for HIV/AIDS have relevance for other specialties and groups of patients within the NHS.

The NHS as a forgetting organization

There were certainly many learning opportunities in the new field of HIV/ AIDS, yet it should be remembered that the culture of the host organization processing this new issue also contained some important pathologies.

'The learning organization' stream of work in essence relabels and continues some of the messages and values previously apparent in the human relations school of management or the organization development movement. It mixes the descriptive (it is functional for knowledge-based organizations based in uncertain environments to organize in this way) and the normative (it is more ethical or liberating for organizations to organize in this way).

Yet the management style in many public sector organizations of the 1980s moved in a very different direction: towards the hardnosed, the measurement of performance and the imposition of top-down action (Pollitt 1990). There was if anything a move away from a consideration of learning and organizational development as important aspects of legitimate management activity.

Elsewhere we have characterized (Pettigrew et al. 1992: Chapter 9) the NHS of the 1980s as a forgetting rather than a learning organization. In the NHS, 'panics' and 'crises' are legion. It is a management system that features endemic short-termism and over-reaction. Attention suddenly switches from one issue to another in response to ever shifting pressures. This culture of short-term panics may be best seen as an exemplification of symbolic decision making. The panics and decisions associated with them are best seen as ceremonial or as empty promises designed to cool down overexcited lobbies. Moreover, there is no internal labour market, so that managerial staff construct their own careers by moving from post to post. Where turnover is highest (e.g. teaching authorities), the organizational memory may be almost entirely absent.

Example: organizational amnesia in a drugs setting

Cranfield et al. (1992) present a case study of the management of service change in post HIV drugs services in an Inner London Drug Dependency Unit. This setting was characterized as a recurring cycle of intense staff effort, burn out and departure. The rate of both clinical and managerial turnover was extremely high. A condition of organizational amnesia set in and valuable experience was lost. For example, the debate over prescribing of controlled drugs (especially injectables) was discussed without conclusion by a staff grouping unaware that it was rehearsing arguments that had taken place ten years earlier.

Early adaptation to HIV/AIDS

Much early work on organizational change focused on the ways in which organizations may be managed to facilitate adaptation to perceived environmental pressures, or contingencies (Burns and Stalker 1961; Lawrence and Lorsch 1967). Implicit in most of this work is that adaptation is advantageous to the organization and is also readily undertaken by, for example, adopting a requisite structure. However, this view of adaptation as the desirable product of deliberate choice has been increasingly challenged as too simplistic.

Critics argue that adaptive change may be inhibited by environmental factors such as specialization, traditions and established ideas, the 'mind sets' of managers and inadequate information (Morgan 1986: 67–68), to say nothing of the restraining effects of lack of resources (Pfeffer and Salancik 1978). Such views are also supported by numerous empirical studies of decision making, which suggest the pre-eminence of the subjective, the arbitrary, the unintentional and even the irrational in the choices made by managers (for an overview of key findings in the literature see March 1988).

An alternative approach is to focus on how the environment influences organizational change. This emphasizes the importance of forces outside organizational control in triggering action, and does much to reduce the element of determinism in the contingency approach. It is also a more helpful perspective to apply when considering the response of the NHS to HIV/AIDS, clearly an unexpected environmental factor. Nevertheless, there are overtones of Charles Darwin and theories of evolution and natural selection about the concept of adaptation in this context, which would, if the perspective were applied too literally, suggest that the outcome of adaptation is always beneficial.

We certainly would not wish to pre-empt the discussion of the organizational response to HIV/AIDS by assuming at the outset that all developments have been advantageous. We need therefore to take the approach suggested by March (1992), who argues for an extension of the concept of evolution beyond narrow models of natural selection, to encompass process as well as outcome. This allows consideration of the inefficiencies of evolutionary processes as instruments of adaptation, as well as their efficiencies. This makes much more sense when we consider the natural history of the development of services for HIV/AIDS, and the various ways in which people and groups at different levels within the organizations involved tried to adapt appropriately to a completely new situation.

In this section we will consider some of the early reactions to HIV, at individual, group and organizational level. At each level of analysis we will look both at some responses which were tried and discarded as perceptions changed and circumstances altered, and at those that have stood the test of time.

Adaptation in response to perceptions of need

One key factor in adaptation to new circumstances is that people may react differently to the same set of stimuli because of prior conceptions. For instance, individual attitudes towards HIV/AIDS varied, even amongst those considering working on infectious diseases (ID) wards:

> We always say to nurses when they come for interview . . . that there is HIV as well as ID. We always mention it to them . . . some people like it, some people don't. At one time you couldn't get bank nurses because I think they were frightened of it being an ID ward and what you could catch.
>
> (ward sister)

Individuals who did not wish to work on this ward would thus never have the opportunity to react and adapt.

Traditional models of care could also prevent adaptation. Haemophilia services, in particular, have been very resistant to adopting new modes of practice in dealing with their HIV-infected patients. As this comment suggests, many staff continue to view HIV as incidental to the 'main' disease, haemophilia:

> I suppose at this centre we still see haemophilia as the main problem, the haemophiliacs themselves would be more worried about

haemophilia than HIV . . . Our patients see it as something else that
has come along which is part of their life within the hospital.

(health service respondent)

Denying and minimizing the important new problems and changed circumstances imposed on haemophiliac patients by HIV/AIDS in this way
precluded adaptation and learning.

There could also be a credibility problem at a more general organizational level. As we saw in Chapter 5, initial responses to the early reports
of a strange new illness affecting gay men in the USA ranged from disbelief
or indifference, to an almost visionary certainty on the part of a few individuals that the issue was of the utmost importance and required an
early response.

To begin with, those who questioned the relevance of the issue to local
circumstances were in the majority, but over time perceptions changed.
Sometimes this happened as a result of new evidence. For instance, the
discovery of the high prevalence of HIV amongst injecting drug users in
Lothian (Peutherer et al. 1985) changed many people's view of the issue
almost overnight, while increasing patient numbers in some London hospitals
helped to convince the government of the need for extra funding.

On the other hand, evidence was not always required for individuals or
groups to revise their views. As AIDS became a high profile media issue
there were many, initially somewhat sceptical, who found themselves swept
along by the enthusiasm of colleagues who were keen to make a response.
Sometimes this changed perception of the issue persisted, leading to permanent alterations in attitudes and work patterns, so that initial adaptation
may truly be said to have led to learning. In some cases, though, as in the
following example, once HIV had become an everyday fact of life, people
reverted to their former, more questioning stance on the issue.

I suppose I was a bit caught up in the excitement, or panic, or hype
or whatever. That here was a huge problem that we needed to do
something about awfully fast . . . there was that sense of excitement,
of wanting to be there. I'm not sure how healthy that was, looking
back at it.

(health service respondent)

The above example, which concerns the setting up of a local telephone
helpline, is typical of the way in which, as Morgan (1986) suggests, organizations and their members can become enmeshed in cognitive traps.
There was, in fact, an already existing phoneline in the same area, but
there was political pressure to be seen to be doing something about HIV/
AIDS and no-one paused to assess the situation and recognize that, for a
fraction of the cost, the capacity of that existing organization could be
enhanced.

Group processes such as these, in which individuals can become involved, almost against their better judgement, in courses of action based on ideas and enthusiasms rather than objective evidence of need or usefulness, were characterized by Janis (1968), in his examination of disastrous American foreign policy decisions, as 'group think'. It is also characteristic of such processes that the collective judgements made can be, and often are, rejected in the cold light of day. Just as President Kennedy is said to have commented after the Cuban missile crisis that he did not know how they could have been so stupid, so the respondent in the above example expressed his uncertainty of the value of what had been achieved.

Other examples of initial reactions to HIV/AIDS, which have since been questioned, include, at individual level, the action of a public health physician in Manchester in issuing an order to detain a patient with AIDS who was thought to pose a risk to others, and the excessive precautions taken to avoid infection by some individuals dealing with people thought to be infected. A number of the group norms that evolved early on are now losing credibility, such as the antitesting stance taken by many counsellors, or the emphasis in health education on 'embedding' HIV within the general curriculum in schools rather than targeting those most at risk.

At an organizational level, the wisdom of creating centralized specialist units for the treatment and care of HIV-related illness is again under debate. It is now recognized that not only can most treatment regimes for HIV disease be instituted at local level, but that patients may experience great difficulty in travelling for long distances for treatment, something that was concealed while most patients were to be found in the London health authorities. It has also been acknowledged that the sudden massive increase in government ring-fenced funding in response to predictions in the Cox Report (DHSS 1988) of a rapid exponential rise in numbers of people with AIDS did not achieve all that was intended, with many authorities being unable to develop plans rapidly enough to utilize all the available resources:

> In 1989–90 some authorities had difficulty in using their allocations within the financial year: the total reported surplus was £15 million ... Some health authorities have used underspends to overcome deficits on other activities, without approval. In these cases monies have generally had to be repaid to the AIDS budget in subsequent years.
>
> (National Audit Office 1991)

Generalization of adaptive responses

If adaptive reactions are later discredited or reversed, learning is confined to the recognition of what is not beneficial. This may be helpful, but does not necessarily lead to discovery of the most appropriate course of action. However, moving a little further along the temporal continuum we now consider situations in which adaptation may also be seen as more closely allied to, though not the same as, true learning. These are situations when a particular response is reproduced over and over again, and can thus at a very elementary level be seen as being learned, but the behaviour does not generalize to other situations, despite the same basic principles being involved.

Most cognitive psychologists take the view that learning involves a degree of understanding of the rules of response selection, as well as simply reacting to a stimulus (Bruner et al. 1956). Organization theorists also may see learning as a cognitive process. Hedberg (1981) suggests that theories of action or myths and sagas are for organizations what cognitive structures are for individuals, while more recently Huber (1991), in a review of the literature on organizational learning, concludes that the development of more and more varied interpretations of information indicates learning. One particularly clear description of the process (which also has the virtue of avoiding treating organizations as if they were sentient entities), is that written by Simon, as long ago as 1953:

> We recognize that environmental forces mold organizations through the mediation of human minds. The process is a learning process ... [involving] growing insights and successive restructurings of the problem as it appears to the humans dealing with it.

By these criteria, many of the adaptive mechanisms observed in organizations responding to HIV/AIDS cannot be said to represent true learning. For instance, once it became officially accepted that there was a real problem, guidelines on new control of infection policies were hastily drawn up and circulated, but individual interpretation of these guidelines varied from the obsessive to the dismissive. Doctors, for instance, might take full precautions and operate: '... all garbed up with helmets over their heads and radios and goodness knows what' (voluntary sector respondent).

In another situation, however, even those same people might behave quite differently:

> [Doctors] are getting so hot under the collar about all these things, about risks etc. and yet everybody says they are the offenders with the sharps injuries, they are the people who take out the drip, put it on the bed and walk away, so that somebody comes and gets a major needle stick injury ... There is a reluctance of doctors to think of themselves as the same as the rest of the human race. They think that they don't need to have medicals, they don't need to have BCGs, you know, they somehow feel that they are fireproof.
>
> (health service respondent)

Thus the general principles behind infection control policies did not necessarily become sufficiently internalized to ensure that they were reflected in appropriate performance whatever the situation.

There are numerous other examples from the data of responses failing to generalize to other situations. One general manager, after avowing support for educating everyone about HIV, requested that an exhibition on the subject was removed in case it should offend members of the health authority. Doctors in acute units, while frequently paying lip service to the importance of community based care for their patients, were in practice often reluctant to refer to other agencies. The rhetoric of joint working was pervasive, but committees were often less than representative of all those concerned.

It was remarked that many of the changes that had been seen in the nature of HIV/AIDS services were also highly applicable to other chronic/terminal conditions (e.g. oncology). There was, for instance, evidence of a patient-focused approach and of user involvement in a number of HIV/AIDS services. Yet we could find few examples of planned movement of staff so as to spread good practice beyond these relatively small pockets.

Learning ways of responding to HIV/AIDS

Having looked at some early adaptive responses to HIV, we now turn to consider how, over time, particular responses were selected and internalized, or learned.

Much of the early work on 'organizational learning' grew out of psychological theories of learning in the individual as a conditioned response to a stimulus (Tolman 1932; Hull 1943; Skinner 1953). Somewhat later, social learning theorists (Mowrer 1950; Maccoby 1959; Bandura 1974) extended this approach to demonstrate that groups of people can collectively learn patterns of behaviour from one another.

Learning in a new situation tends to be incremental, because the actual process of learning occurs in and through individuals, but a particular perception of and response to an issue can come to be shared by a number of people and ultimately throughout an organization. So organizational learning can occur at three levels. Shared understanding can occasionally be achieved simultaneously by large numbers of people (for instance, when an earthquake occurs), but normally a collective perception develops through individuals emerging as early learners. That learning may then diffuse outwards from them, first to their immediate groups and networks, and then to the larger organizations of which these are a part.

Time is a key element in this process, for, while individuals, particularly if motivated, may learn relatively quickly; the diffusion of that learning to groups takes longer, and to create shared understanding at organizational level may take longer still. Of course, group or organizational learning may never happen at all if the organizational context is not receptive (Pettigrew et al. 1992), but even where the ground is fertile, the sharing of information is a time-consuming business. As Cangelosi and Dill (1965) pointed out, the subgroups within which the learning processes initially take place may not possess good systems for communicating at an organizational level.

So how have individuals, groups and organizations learned to deal with the HIV/AIDS issue within DHAs? Individuals learn when motivated by the prospect of external or internal reward, but learning may also occur without conscious intention through being exposed to a range of environmental influences, either deliberately or unintentionally.

As we have seen in previous chapters, our case study material provides examples of all these. Individual professional autonomy enabled doctors from such diverse specialties as immunology, genitourinary medicine, infectious diseases, haematology and public health medicine to pursue internally generated interest in HIV/AIDS. 'Product champions' (Stocking 1985, Ferlie and Pettigrew 1990) emerged as an important focus for service development. The prospect of rewards in the form of resources prompted even those with no initial interest to learn about the issue in order to make credible bids for extra staff or new equipment. Apart from this instrumental motivation, there was also a strong involvement from clinical academics who could well be creating new knowledge about the disease through their research projects. Such actors could be committed to research and knowledge generation as an end in itself.

Environmental cues also influenced learning. Yellow 'BioHazard' stickers took on new significance with the advent of HIV/AIDS and staff learned to take extra safety precautions. Office walls covered in explicit posters assisted people to learn about and become familiar with the social and cultural aspects of HIV/AIDS.

Experiential, formal, informal and coincidental learning

The literature on organizational change suggests that much learning comes about as a result of experience (for a review see Huber 1991). Certainly much of the early learning about HIV/AIDS within DHAs was individual and experiential: clinicians learned from experience the combinations of drugs best suited to unusual infections, and technicians learned to use new HIV tests by practising laboratory techniques (Bennett et al. 1990). Key clinicians and community medicine specialists also made a deliberate effort to try to inform staff and pre-empt any anxiety on their part, once something was known about the nature of the virus and the routes of transmission:

I spent a lot of time, as did other members of the group, going round giving talks to hospital staff in this hospital, every hospital, time and time again. It got rather tedious, but it was much appreciated I know, and I think people felt a lot more secure as a result of that.

Once HIV/AIDS was recognized as a policy issue, there was further emphasis and resources put into formal training. Staff attended lectures and seminars on clinical aspects of the syndrome and on new techniques of infection control and patient care.

However, a formal approach to learning about HIV/AIDS was sometimes insufficient to help people deal with deep seated anxieties or feelings. There was a need for an 'unlearning' (Hedberg 1981) of some traditional values and attitudes if patients were to be treated with sensitivity, but AIDS is a highly charged issue and some people's perceptions were slow to change. Early initiatives, for example, attempted to calm fears of health care staff about the risk of infection, but there were still many examples of staff at all levels reacting with excessive caution. The most successful formal training programmes have been constructed to address, not just the need to learn new techniques, but the more fundamental requirement to change attitudes and value systems.

In every intentional learning situation, there is also the possibility for unintentional learning. Most people remember the 'gravestones and icebergs' TV commercials, but both have been criticized for unintentionally making people so frightened of AIDS that they blocked out the message (Brandt 1988). Some commercials about drug use have been said to reinforce stereotypes and stigmatize drug users. Mixed messages could also be a problem. Training programmes emphasized that HIV could not be transmitted through ordinary social contact, but at ward level plates and cutlery used by people with HIV were sometimes handled separately from those used by other patients.

Consideration of the learning processes precipitated by a particular stimulus tends to focus attention on responses relating specifically to that issue. However, another aspect of organizational learning that may be forgotten is that the organizational response to one issue may trigger learning in relation to a cluster of other issues, only loosely connected to the initial precipitating stimulus. This process might be termed coincidental learning.

Brown and Duguid (1991) give a number of examples of how difficult it may be for organizations to make the conceptual leap required to 'reregister' their environments, and how a novel stimulus may be effective in instigating procedural change in organizations 'trapped in their own world view'. In just this way HIV/AIDS, while itself requiring the acquisition of new techniques, skills, values and attitudes, has also been the catalyst for forcing reappraisal of some more global issues of policy:

HIV and AIDS, it's actually been a dose of anti-freeze in the radiator, its coming out of the holes and its showing up holes across the board in the health and social services . . . So what HIV in the radiator has done is to show what is bad practice.

(social services respondent)

Such matters as allowing people to choose their treatment and care regimes, supplying sterile injecting equipment to drug users rather than pursuing an ideal of total abstinence, protecting confidentiality and controlling cross-infection, were not new to HIV/AIDS. What was new was that suddenly these issues were being debated in the full glare of public and media scrutiny, compelling management attention and ultimately new working practices where before they had been low on the list of priorities.

Thus, dealing with HIV/AIDS has prompted coincidental organizational learning on a wide range of topics and issues, which might otherwise have remained unaddressed.

The NHS – becoming a learning organization?

It is paradoxical that the NHS – which is a classic example of a knowledge- and education-based organization – exhibits a culture which seems to make organizational learning difficult rather than easy.

Following on from a consideration of the different forms of *reactive* learning, it is thus pertinent to ask whether AIDS has been deliberately, or proactively, used as a vehicle for more general organizational learning within the NHS. A higher level capacity for organizational learning has been seen by Normann (1985) as one way in which organizations can improve their ability to manage successive strategic change processes by creating a form of organization better able to respond to continuing environmental change. This has similarities with Argyris and Schon's (1978) concept of 'double loop' rather than 'single loop' learning, whereby organizations not only learn to cope with a particular change but more generically learn how to learn.

Often the processes by which organizations develop a capacity to learn have remained surprisingly unexplored in the literature. Jones and Hendry (1992) ask the important question: how is a learning organization created? They suggest that triggers may include the following events and situations:

- The need to get greater participation from the work force.
- Producing better products/services in more efficient ways.
- The arrival of a new chair who wants to change the culture of the organization.

- Government intervention (e.g. issuing of charter of rights).
- Perception of a growing performance gap.
- When management experiences a shift in their own perception about the value of people.

The arrival of unheralded issues such as HIV/AIDS might be thought to be another trigger for the construction of a learning organization as they require new forms of knowledge to be generated, practice to be overhauled and mechanisms constructed for the management of gross uncertainty.

More concretely, we can ask: has the response to HIV/AIDS prompted a greater use of more minimalistic structures such as problem-solving groups and *ad hoc* task forces (Hedberg et al. 1976)? Is there a more self-conscious strategic process? Are there innovations in planning methodology away from formal long-range plans and towards the scripting-in of uncertainty?

The answers to these questions cannot be unequivocal. Organizational development was in any case a theme – if only a secondary theme – in the NHS of the mid-1980s. At this very general level, a district general manager in one of our case study authorities, for instance, argued – outside the specific context of HIV/AIDS – that learning to cope with change was a major issue for general management:

> It was recognized from an early stage that one of the key management challenges was not just to implement change, but to develop an organization's capacity to cope with change. The aim, in a sense, was to create a different kind of organization, capable of learning, responding to and even creating change, rather than simply reacting to it.

However, the key feature of HIV/AIDS, which distinguished it from many other change issues in the health service, was that changes in the nature of the issue tended to be rapid, unpredictable and looked likely to continue indefinitely. With little hard information available, predictions of likely numbers of patients varied, sometimes almost on a daily basis, and certainly according to which epidemiologist or clinician was talking at the time. Resources to fund HIV/AIDS were at first so slender as to force concerned doctors to use media publicity to trigger governmental action. Then suddenly, in 1989–90, the allocation was increased to such an extent that health authorities found it nearly impossible to arrange to spend all they were given in the time available. Even at a clinical level changes in knowledge about AIDS and how to treat it were so rapid that patients were sometimes as well informed as their doctors and the old 'doctor knows best' approach proved difficult to sustain:

> Most major discoveries are now not published, or they are subsequently, but they're not published in the medical journals, they're published in newspapers. That puts us at a big disadvantage

... Whereas you can read the *BMJ* and the *New England Journal of Medicine* every week, at least know what's in it and look for things like that. You can't read all the papers every day and the magazines and the women's magazines carry all this as well. So it becomes almost impossible to maintain the feeling normally that you have, that you actually know more than the patients, when sometimes you actually don't.

(consultant physician)

A useful analogy may be made with the requirement for continuing rather than one-off innovation in the electronics industry, where Jelinek and Schoonhoven (1990) have argued:

The story of electronics is not of a one shot or two shot battle, but of an ongoing barrage of change that shows every sign of continuing indefinitely. Success lies not in pulling it off once, but in creating a self sustaining organizational system that will replicate technological innovation repeatedly over the long run.

There was some evidence that HIV/AIDS, coming at the same time as general management, could be used as a useful test bed for building a new type of organization outside the usual hierarchies. In one of our authorities a general manager said:

It was quite a good illustration of the way a problem can be now more effectively handled as a planning and management issue. Under general management, I had the facility without any formal sanction from the District Management Board other than 'you have got a brief: AIDS', to pull together the right sort of people to carry forward that particular task, and pull in where I felt I could get the right financial help and the right service help.

Interestingly, the next major change issue which this group had to address was their reaction to the introduction of the quasi market, and the split between purchasers and providers. The health authority as a whole was seen as adapting slowly, but HIV/AIDS was one of a small minority of services seen as keen and as a 'fast mover.' The good prehistory, the self-contained nature of the service groupings, the presence of a strategy group and of a specialist senior registrar in charge of planning, were all seen as contributing to this rapid pace of learning. Here was some evidence of a group 'learning how to learn'. However, it proved difficult to replicate this approach on other HIV/AIDS groups set up within the authority: only the original group seemed to have developed this generic competence to learn.

Such an outcome was, however, unusual, and the overall verdict must be one of disappointment. The general manager quoted was the exception rather than the rule, and in most of our sites general managers did not take a particular interest in HIV/AIDS, seeing it as an issue for public health. Hence generic management theories, which some of the new managers were utilizing as they set up new systems elsewhere within health authorities, were less likely to be seen as applicable to HIV; while the special machinery which was often set up for HIV/AIDS was rarely linked to such explicit theories of action and was vulnerable to 'normalization' when the sense of immediate crisis faded.

As we have noted above, the reorganization of the NHS and the development of an internal market in healthcare has provided a number of opportunities for management of HIV/AIDS to offer a model for the new purchaser/provider culture. For instance, alone amongst specialties, the money for HIV/AIDS was ring-fenced and the money spent had to be accounted for annually in the AIDS Control Act Reports. In theory this should have allowed those running the services to have a much clearer view of the relationship between resources and service provision than did most other management teams prior to the implementation of the NHS reforms. Unfortunately, however, a lack of investment in setting up good information systems has meant that in many cases those with responsibility for planning services have not had appropriate financial information available. Indeed, when interviewed, some Chairs of AIDS Advisory Committees had no idea who held the budget, how it was allocated, and expenditure to date in the current year. Some committees did make strenuous efforts to obtain such information, but found themselves up against treasurer's departments, which had not been used to accounting specifically for small portions of their budget, and were loath to expose their systems for robbing Peter to pay Paul.

Thus, far from being able to provide a prototype for a newly cost-aware NHS, HIV services in general were sucked into an old financial system in which individual departments and specialties generally had little to do with, and knew very little about the financial consequences of their activity. This eventually caused great concern when, in 1990, the National Audit Office was commissioned by the government to examine the arrangements for the planning, funding and provision of health services in response to the HIV epidemic. The report (National Audit Office 1991) was unequivocal in stating the inadequacy of the financial data:

> To target resources towards treatment and care, the Department need an accurate estimate of the resources used in providing services for those with HIV and AIDS. In most districts the necessary costing and activity data were not readily available ... The Department acknowledges that the systems for allocating resources may be crude.

The report goes on to suggest that the introduction of contracting should make resource allocation and assumed activity levels more explicit. This is another interesting comment, as in most authorities the multidisciplinary approach to service development, coupled with most of the money being allocated to the health service, had meant that numerous services, particularly in the voluntary sector, had been funded on what was actually a contractual basis, though frequently without the individual elements of those services being formally specified.

With fixed sums of money available, and discrete, newly developed services for a relatively small patient population, we would argue that HIV services were in a splendid position to have been in the vanguard of the new contracting arrangements. However, in most cases, those managing the services failed to perceive this as an opportunity for developing new management systems as well as innovative responses to the task. Instead they adopted the *ad hoc* approach, without adequate systems for monitoring process and evaluating outcome, which has characterized so much service development in the NHS in the past.

In consequence, rather than the new circumstances precipitating new management arrangements, the Department of Health has been forced to acknowledge that the rudimentary information systems currently available are inadequate to support formal purchasing arrangements for HIV services. Thus implementation of contracting, planned to start in 1992, has been deferred for at least a year and possibly longer, and HIV services will, in fact, be the laggards in the new purchaser/provider culture.

Concluding discussion

In this chapter we have used the example of HIV/AIDS to explore the theme of adaptation and learning. The first part of the chapter considered some of the processes of adaptation by which the people, groups and organizations studied responded to HIV/AIDS. This argued that some initial 'knee-jerk' reactions were shown to be non-adaptive and were later abandoned, whereas others were seen as appropriate and, over time, became internalized. We have also suggested that some of this behaviour has become sufficiently permanent and widespread to be characterized as 'learned behaviour', although much of this learning took place at an individual and group level rather than across the whole organization. In the last section we explored the meaning of the concept of a 'learning organization', and asked if the NHS, in its response to HIV/AIDS, can be considered to merit such an appellation. Despite some interesting exceptions, we were in general sceptical as to whether much had been achieved in this direction.

Although we use the term 'organizational learning' as a convenient shorthand for learning which is collectively disseminated and internalized, we of course recognize that this term is, as Argyris and Schon (1978) point out, merely a metaphor, and that in fact 'members of the organization act as learning agents for the organization'.

In this discussion section, we now need to ask whether the reaction of the health authorities studied to this particular, and some would argue unique, issue can have relevance for increasing our understanding of the learning process in organizations. Can anything be inferred from the response to HIV/AIDS about general mechanisms by which learning takes place, factors that promote and inhibit learning and of how organizations may take a proactive approach towards organizational transformation through learning, i.e. towards becoming a 'learning organization'?

First, we need to consider the possible argument that HIV/AIDS is too specific an issue for generalizations to be made from it. In some ways, of course, this is bound to be true, but in this it is no different from any other individual issue that may trigger learning. There are certainly aspects of HIV that cannot be compared with any other current health issue, although, as we have seen in earlier chapters, some comparisons may be made with diseases that had a higher profile some years ago, such as tuberculosis and syphilis, which also raised social and moral, as well as purely medical, issues. However, we are suggesting in this chapter that much, if not most, organizational learning is derived from responses made to particular stimuli, rather than *a priori* from deliberate intent to learn. It therefore seems safe to conclude that, whatever the particular features of an issue, there are also likely to be some commonalities. What then, can HIV illuminate about some general mechanisms of organizational learning?

To begin with, we can look at how well the data on HIV supports other empirical evidence concerning processes of organizational learning. The view of early theorists in psychology – that learning comes about as a response to a particular stimulus or stimuli – has never been seriously questioned, and the main conceptual leap made by management theorists was to suggest that this theory could explain collective as well as individual action. Different writers have given different names to the various types of learning process. March and Olsen (1976), for instance, stayed with the psychological terminology for their model of the organizational learning cycle as a stimulus–response system, Argyris and Schon (1978) identify single-loop and double-loop learning, Hedberg (1981) uses the terms defensive and offensive adjustment while Huber (1991) suggests that at least five separate types of process are involved. All these, however, explain similar phenomena, and we have preferred here to settle for a very simple typology, making a distinction only between learning as reactive and proactive processes.

On this basis, the data on HIV provide many examples of reactive learning that show parallels with observations made of learning processes around other subjects and in other settings. There have been examples of both adaptive and non-adaptive 'knee-jerk' reactions to a sudden and unexpected environmental stimulus. We have traced the process of learning about HIV from a few early enthusiasts 'sensing' that something new was emerging and passing on that learning to the wider groups of which they were a part. We have also seen examples of 'unlearning' (Hedberg 1981) traditional ways of working and attitudes to different groups of patients, in response to environmental pressures towards consumerism and 'alternative' forms of therapy.

Additionally, examination of learning processes in relation to HIV has highlighted the importance of informal as distinct from formal learning. Here the evidence suggests that formal training programmes, so beloved of most major organizations whether in the public or private sector, may not be nearly so effective in actually altering behaviour as people believe, particularly if what is to be learned is not purely factual, but requires people to change their fundamental beliefs and attitudes. Also highlighted have been the effects of environmental stimuli in producing changes in behaviour.

Early on in this chapter, the point was made that learning should be recognized as an explicitly temporal process. This is something that may be glossed over by those more concerned with the process itself, but it may be essential to place organizational learning around a particular issue in the context of other changing elements and differing time frames both within and without the organization. Studying the learning process around HIV makes this particularly clear, for only by locating it within its ten-year time frame can the different dynamics that have affected the process be understood. HIV in Britain arose in the climate of a swing towards traditional moral values as expressed in Thatcherite ideology, and new moves towards managerialism and monetary restrictions within the NHS. All these tended to affect attitudes and values and initially slowed the learning process. On the other hand, HIV also arose in a climate that, at least by rhetoric, celebrated consumer choice, entrepreneurialism and personal autonomy, all tending to encourage the adoption of new attitudes and working practices.

We conclude that, at least in terms of the ability to learn, the NHS as a whole seems so much less than the sum of its parts. It is a knowledge- and education-based organization; it contains an important research component, including clinical academics engaged in cutting-edge research (some of whom went on to 'sense' the HIV/AIDS issue and became early product champions in our case studies) and energetic and 'intelligent' (e.g. concerned to gather information from a variety of external quarters) small groups formed around the HIV/AIDS issue. All these factors, one might have thought, would have contributed to an active concern to stimulate learning at an organizational level.

Yet diffusion of learning outside these individuals and groupings proved problematic. Moreover, there was little evidence that the response might have been usefully mined from an organizational development point of view as a naturally occurring experiment. Over time, organizational responses have routinized and decision-making machinery has been subject to a process of 'normalization.' As an organization, the NHS seems still to forget more than it learns.

CHAPTER

9
_____

Concluding discussion and a look into the future

Overview of the main findings

In this final chapter, we take an overview of the findings that have emerged from the preceding empirical chapters. What have we learnt about the organizational and managerial response to HIV/AIDS that we did not know before? What general themes have been illuminated by the data presented?

In the second part of the chapter, we liberate ourselves from data, taking a more speculative look at the future and discussing which challenges may lie ahead for the management of HIV/AIDS services in the next five or ten years. We conclude by outlining some areas where future theoretical work could fruitfully be concentrated.

The evidence presented suggests a much messier, inchoate and emergent innovation process than contained within many of the prescriptive management of change models (e.g. Ottaway 1976; Nadler 1983). One is struck by the diverse and highly pluralist nature of the leadership process with SMOs, 'bureaucratic insurgents' and clinical product champions playing key roles. While individuals were important as innovators – particularly in the earliest stages – as the issue grew in scope and complexity, so the formation of small teams and interorganizational coalitions became a prerequisite for effective management.

On the other hand, we found general managers, with a few notable exceptions, taking something of a back seat. Perhaps this was because

HIV/AIDS was perceived, particularly at the beginning, as primarily a clinical issue. Managers became briefly interested when it became clear that there were (adverse or favourable) financial implications, and sometimes, in later stages, had a significant controlling or damping effect (Ferlie and Pettigrew 1990), but there is little evidence of the managerial grouping as a whole playing a creative or developmental role.

The process of change can only be fully understood through the use of a longitudinal approach to analysis. Important parts of the historical antecedents that shaped the response – such as the Contagious Diseases Acts – went back to the last century. Alongside bursts of change, therefore, stood strong streams of continuity.

Change was emergent more than managed. Programmatic interventions or designated 'change managers' were conspicuous by their absence, though change management might be seen to have been implicit in the brief given to some of the early coordinators brought in from the voluntary sector. Neither was there explicit 'transition planning'; rather events unfolded. It is clear that the history, culture and micropolitics of the organization have to be taken fully into account in understanding precisely how services developed in each locality. The evidence presented is more consistent with Mintzberg's (1989) concept of an emergent rather than a planned process of strategic change.

This is not to say that no pattern could be discerned in the process and that each case study is *sui generis*. In fact a number of linking themes were identified, which help us understand variations in the process across the localities studied.

The role of ideology in shaping perceptions

Although the response to all change issues is modified by how they are perceived by key actors, with HIV/AIDS the role played by ideological perspectives in both interpreting the issue and mediating action was unusually visible, and played a central part in our analysis of the issue. It was indeed the 'construction of reality' (Berger and Luckmann 1966) rather than objective evidence that was important, from the epidemiology to the need for service development, and those who were good at presentation had the edge over those who were not.

Over time, some ideological perspectives have seemed to be taking precedence. For instance, pejorative, moralistic terms such as 'addict' or 'drug *mis*user' have been largely replaced by the more innocuous 'drug *user*'. It is no longer 'politically correct' to talk of homosexuals, or AIDS 'victims', nor to be visibly shocked when faced with explicit health promotion material that, in other settings, might be seen as pornographic. Such changes seem to have come about through acceptance by those espousing a liberal ideology of many of the values vigorously promoted by radical social movements. However, there is a question about how much people's attitudes have really changed or whether a more conservative 'moral majority' view has merely gone underground for the present, only to re-emerge if and when conditions become more favourable.

The role of change agents

Clinical product champions

Consistent with the findings of other studies in both industrial (Rothwell 1976) and health care (Stocking 1985) settings, we noted the key role of individual product champions (often clinicians or clinical academics) in supporting the innovation process. Despite the introduction of general management, clinical and research 'segments' continued to form around HIV/AIDS in an unpredictable fashion (Bucher and Stelling 1977) and early clinical product champions could emerge from these segments.

The clinical product champions were the early learners who for a variety of reasons picked up the issue and ran with it, transmitting their energy, enthusiasm and knowledge to others both directly and through symbolic activity of various kinds. As well as energy and personality, such clinical product champions – in order to be fully effective – needed team building skills, diplomatic skills and a sound organizational power base from which to operate.

Representatives of social movements and social movement organizations

We noted the important role of social movements, SMOs and attendant ideologies in a number of the localities studied. Some theorists of social movements have seen them as sectarian and backward-looking, unable to play an effective decision-making role in advanced societies (Touraine 1981). We, on the other hand, found that people with an ideological commitment to, for instance, 'gay and lesbian rights' or 'alternative medicine' had some success in capturing the specialist HIV labour market being set up inside the NHS, in effect acting as 'bureaucratic insurgents' from within.

Perhaps surprisingly, we found that SMOs tended to take a relatively 'inclusive' stance in the management of relations with their environment. Zealots were less in evidence than diplomats, and hearts were not always worn on sleeves. Perhaps this could be linked with the emergence of a paid salariat in both public and voluntary sector settings. Radical critics (e.g. Patton 1990) complain precisely of this drift away from the initial charismatic base towards formalization and bureaucratization. AIDS service organizations now exhibit a high degree of dependence on government funding. Perhaps in reaction against this general trend towards cooptation, new and more radical 'groupuscules' (e.g. ACT UP) have emerged, which retain many of the features of an SMO as an organizational form.

As one would expect in a field of ideologized change, the symbolic and cultural aspects of the HIV/AIDS issue were indeed found to be of major importance, but they were only rarely self-consciously undertaken by change agents. This was clearly evident in the construction of a collective acceptable language system. Such a language system emerged organically from a particular subculture, later to be codified by official bodies. We would question whether such symbolic aspects are likely to represent tractable management material, especially as many different symbolic systems were mobilized by the HIV/AIDS issue.

The organizational effects of crisis

There is a debate apparent in the literature between those who argue that the presence of a crisis exerts a debilitating effect on management and those who see it as an energising force. Clearly this question is of great relevance to the processing of the HIV/AIDS issue, given its construction as a national crisis in 1986–87.

Our evidence suggested a three-phase model of crisis management: (1) in the short term there was evidence of 'epidemic psychology', with waves of panic, fear, guilt and the periodic occurrence of untoward incidents; (2) in the medium term, there was found to be an explosion of energy, mobilization and joint purpose around the issue; but (3) in the long term there was a danger of burn-out and of issue succession.

Joint working

Because of the multiplicity of organizations and settings involved, securing joint working was a major theme in the management of HIV/AIDS services. We found on the whole that mandated cooperation and formal structures by themselves had little impact. However, certain informal organizational processes acted as important facilitators (as well as inhibitors) of joint working.

Small joint groups were of particular importance. Many of these were set up very early on by those responsible for 'championing' the issue and were notable for their inclusivity. Later, when such groups became mandatory, it was notable that there was a drift towards either becoming big and unwieldy, as more and more interest groups provided representatives or to membership becoming dominated by the health service (this was particularly evident as groups reconfigured into purchasing bodies).

Learning processes

Finally, we highlighted the informal and experiential side of much individual and small group learning. A formal approach to learning about

HIV/AIDS sometimes offered little help in dealing with deep-seated anxieties or feelings. At a wider level, the impact of educational initiatives was not always predictable, leading to unintentional messages being received along with the intentional ones.

In terms of the NHS as a whole, we were pessimistic about the extent to which the lessons learned from HIV/AIDS were likely to generalize to other related issues. It seemed that sustained organizational learning had yet to take place, and that obvious parallels with needs evident in other service settings had not been drawn. The NHS, it appears, may still be more of a forgetting than a learning organization.

Receptivity for innovation – a discussion

In our previous work (Pettigrew et al. 1992), we explained variation in the rate and pace of strategic service change observed in a sample of DHAs across a number of health care issues through the use of the metaphor of receptive and non-receptive contexts for change. The fieldwork for this earlier study was carried out between 1986 and 1990.

The evidence collected during the later HIV/AIDS study can be used to test our original model. Are our early findings confirmed, developed or refuted as a result of this later evidence? The more they are confirmed, the greater the probability that the model captures some general principles of organizational change – at least within health care organizations – which generalize across issues and time periods. Conversely, the more the early findings are refuted, the greater the evidence that change processes in health care are shaped by highly idiosyncratic factors, which vary unpredictably from one issue and from one time period to another.

The original study identified eight 'signs and symptoms' of receptivity, which seemed to be associated with a faster pace of change. We outline each in turn and then assess the significance of the evidence coming from the HIV/AIDS studies. We also – and this is an addition to the work undertaken in the first study – try to accord a temporal ordering to the features identified. Some can be seen as present during the whole of the change process, while others only came on stream later on.

Feature 1: Environmental pressure – intensity, scale and orchestration

While studies outside the NHS (Pettigrew 1985) have highlighted the significant role of intense and large-scale environmental pressure in triggering periods of radical change, the picture in the NHS is more complex as in some instances excessive short term pressure can deflect or drain energy out of the system. In other cases, environmental pressure can produce movement, perhaps where it is moderate or stable in nature, or where the pressure is skilfully orchestrated (the importance of subjectivity was confirmed in our material on the issue recognition process in HIV/AIDS). In our first study, many of the crises were financial in nature, and while they could produce areas of movement in some localities, in others they led to denial, scapegoating and a collapse of decision-making routines.

The evidence from the HIV/AIDS case studies clearly points to the greater and more consistent force of a perceived external crisis in triggering radical organizational development. Here was a health care issue rather than a financial issue. Here also was an issue with a high media profile, bottom up pressure from external social movement organizations, and (by 1986) top-down pressure from central government for local action.

The response to HIV/AIDS can be seen as an example of crisis management in almost its purest form. In this extreme manifestation, it seems to approximate more to some earlier studies of organizational change in the private sector (Pettigrew 1985) than did our earlier NHS findings, which instead highlighted the role of continuing, moderate and stable financial pressure in triggering organizational change in some localities. The importance of orchestrating a sense of crisis as a trigger for change was, however, as clearly evident in the HIV/AIDS case studies as in our previous study.

Feature 2: The fit between the change agenda and the locale

Previous research on, for example, human resource change has indicated that various features of the locale where change is to occur may inhibit or accelerate change. Thus Hardy's (1985) study of organizational closure demonstrates how and why climate building for such changes is linkable to high levels of unemployment, and consequential changes in the power balance between managers and trade unionists.

Our first study on change in the NHS also indicated that the nature of the locale had an impact on how easy it was to achieve change, for example, whether there is a teaching hospital presence, the strength and nature of the local political culture and the degree of unionization and militancy of the local NHS workforce.

With regard to HIV/AIDS services, we would point to three features of the locale that can be seen as particularly important. The first refers to the strength or weakness of local SMOs. Clearly there are vast differences between Inner London and some rural areas, and these differences affected the dynamics of service development.

The second refers to the differences between radical/liberal and conservative local political cultures. This was not simply a crude party split, but refers to the nature of local political regimes: some Labour cities were in fact highly nervous of action in this field, while some traditionalist Conservative London boroughs were active and supportive.

We would thirdly highlight the presence/absence of a teaching hospital. On the credit side, a teaching hospital will bring with it academic medicine, with a tradition of service development on the back of 'soft' research funding. Also, pragmatically, the specialties concerned with HIV/AIDS tended to be concentrated in teaching authorities. On the other hand, a highly professionalized ethos may sometimes crowd out social movement activity, at least at a strategic level.

Both the first two features – environmental pressure and the suitability of the locale – can be seen as part of the inheritance and as largely exogenous to the system. We now move on to consider features that are more related to action and choice.

Feature 3: A supportive organizational culture

'Organizational culture' is a currently fashionable term and remains a fascinating, but difficult, topic to study. 'Culture' refers to deep-seated assumptions and values far below surface manifestations, officially espoused ideologies or even patterns of behaviour. The invisible barrier of culture may cause myopia and inertia within organizations and a supportive organizational culture may be about challenging and changing assumptions and beliefs.

In our first study, it was not possible to talk about a single NHS culture, but rather we found a collection of different subcultures which may inhabit the same locale (e.g. managerial, clinical). We particularly focused on the managerial subculture and put forward a number of features as being associated with a high rate of change.

The importance of organizational culture was confirmed in the HIV/AIDS study, although we were here often dealing with an issue-based rather than a role-based or institution-based subculture (e.g. general management or the teaching hospital). There were clear differences found between the issue subculture and the culture of the host organization – it emerged as a separate microclimate.

Much of this culture originated in voluntary sector SMOs (where it had, as we discuss in Chapter 4, a strong ideological component) and spread throughout HIV/AIDS services, leading to a culture characterized by strong norms of 'correct' behaviour towards those affected by HIV/AIDS. 'Culture' was thus found to be a powerful analytic device, much more so than traditional concern with formal structure. There was a need for the culture to be inclusive rather than exclusive, and able to handle the crossing of boundaries. The evidence suggested – perhaps surprisingly – that this was often the case. The development of a shared HIV culture including clinicians, managers and SMOs was found to be highly energizing and facilitated interorganizational cooperation.

As in the last study, we saw the importance of such cultural features as: flexibility in patterns of working (e.g. *ad hoc* task forces); role blur-ring; openness to innovation and experimentation; support for research, development and evaluation; a positive self-image and a sense of past success.

Feature 4: Availability of key people leading change

Another important feature identified in the last study was the availability of key people in critical posts leading change. We did not here refer to heroic and individualistic 'macho managers', but found that leadership was exercized in a much more subtle and pluralist way. The small group – as well as the single individual – could be an effective vehicle, so con-scious team building could be important with selectors.

A diversity of leadership was apparent both in terms of its occupational base (clinicians as well as managers) and hierarchical level (junior as well as senior staff). It was also found that often personalities rather than posts were important: personal skills were more important in managing change than formal status or rank within the organization. These findings were consistent with the results of recent research (Pettigrew and Whipp 1991) and writing (Nadler and Tushman 1990) on private sector strategic change processes, which pointed to the need to broaden and deepen the leadership cadre.

The previous finding that leadership within the NHS was a multilayered and pluralist activity was confirmed and strengthened in the study of HIV/ AIDS services, but there were differences in the cast of actors. By them-selves, individual general managers played a secondary role. Although clinical product champions represented the clearest individual focus in the earliest stages of the response, a wider range of people quickly became mobilized in our localities, and over time we identified the increasing role of small teams and especially of more diffuse networks in facilitating change. We see an even greater importance of the network as a mode of organizing in this study as compared to our previous findings.

Feature 5: Simplicity and clarity of goals and priorities

This focusing issue arises from the conclusion in our first study that managers varied greatly in their ability to narrow down the change agenda into a set of key priorities, and to insulate the core from the constantly shifting short term pressures apparent in the NHS. The danger was that the number of 'priorities' would escalate until they became meaningless. Rather, persistence and patience in the pursuit of objectives over a long period seemed to be associated with achieving strategic change. Skills in complexity and conflict reduction could also be important here, in trying to contain complex problems in simpler organizational frameworks.

Of course, HIV/AIDS represents a single issue, and as such must be seen as narrower in scope than the multi-issue analysis we undertook in the first study. It was also perhaps different in that service development was assisted by the sense of 'mission' developed by many of those closely involved in the process. We did indeed find evidence of 'managerial butterflies' who moved in and out of the change process, and did not demonstrate sustained interest and commitment, and there were those who could be seen as 'using' HIV/AIDS to gain a toe-hold on the career ladder. Against this, many of the early clinical product champions can be seen as staying with the issue, and (perhaps surprisingly) not showing evidence of 'burn-out'. Although specialists demonstrate other disadvantages, they may have the advantage of 'stickability', if only pragmatically because they find it difficult to move onto alternative issues.

Feature 6: Cooperative interorganizational networks

In our first study, many changes in the priority group sector in particular were underscored by the development and management of interorganizational networks with such agencies as social services departments and voluntary organizations. Health authorities had little power in these settings, but rather had to win influence. A number of features could enrich these networks, such as a system of financial incentives, clear referral and communication points, shared ideologies or history and the existence of boundary spanners who crossed agency divides.

The most effective networks were found to be informal but also purposeful (rather than self-absorbed and narcissistic) however – as the consequence of the personalities and not posts argument – they were also fragile and vulnerable to turnover. One director of social services might be interested in mental handicap; the next in the elderly. However at their best such networks provided an opportunity for trading and education, for commitment and energy raising and for marrying top-down and bottom-up concerns.

The importance of this finding was confirmed in the HIV/AIDS study where the NHS, social services and the voluntary sector could all be seen as having a key role in the provision of service. The effective crossing of such boundaries was a key management skill. We found once more that the most powerful shapers of joint working were informal rather than formal: mandated cooperation by itself had little impact. We highlighted the particularly important role of the small joint group and of the ideologized network.

Feature 7: Effective managerial/clinical relations

The nature of the managerial/clinical interface was found to be critically important in our first study. The pattern found was one of wide variation in the quality of such relations, and when clinicians had gone into opposition, they could exert a powerful block on change. Managers varied in the extent to which they saw relationship-building and trading with clinicians as a core part of their brief.

Manager/clinician relations were easier where negative stereotypes had broken down. For managers, it was important to understand what clinicians valued, and hence what they had to do to engage in effective trading relations. From the clinical perspective, there was found to be an important group of clinicians – who had often come up through the medical advisory machinery – who think more managerially and strategically. Such strategic clinicians were critical people for management to identify and foster.

The importance of this earlier finding was confirmed in this study in a small number of high prevalence authorities where resource flows had been built up at an early date. Here general managers took on a resource controlling role from an early date (1986), forcing the question of clinical/ managerial relationships. In other localities, however, this feature had been less noticeable in the past but was emerging as an issue for the future as the management of AIDS services became increasingly systematized (e.g. emergence of purchaser roles, of clinical directors and of business managers). We suspect that this feature will be of rising importance in the future.

We also noted the importance of the role of medical managers, such as public health physicians, who were active in some authorities from very early on, and in most from 1986, when the government required the appointment of a 'nominated physician' to cover the HIV/AIDS issue. Some of these have proved very successful in tempering the 'empire-building' tendencies of clinical colleagues and promoting a model of community, rather than acute sector, care. Others, however, have been less interested and less sucessful, leaving the field to the clinicians to configure services.

Feature 8: The quality and coherence of 'policy'

As well as the managerial process involved, the quality of 'policy' generated at a local level was found to be an important factor in mediating change in the first study. Analytically, the possession of data played a major role in substantiating a solid case, especially in convincing scientific publics, and we would not generally support the argument of 'paralysis by analysis' (Peters and Waterman 1982). The ordering of such data within clear conceptual thinking helped frame highly uncertain strategic issues, with the most robust strategies also considering questions of coherence between goals, feasibility and implementation requirements and the need to complement service strategies with other functional strategies (such as finance or human resources). A broad vision seemed more likely to generate movement than a blueprint, and to have significant process and implementation benefits in terms of commitment-building and allowing interest groups to buy into the change process, allowing top-down pressure to be married with bottom-up concern.

This initial finding can be developed in the light of the later HIV/AIDS study. In the early years central policy guidance was very loose, with the result that interested localities had the opportunity to develop their own strategic frameworks. This was particularly important in the highest prevalence localities, where substantial government funding was made available early on because of real concerns – not later realized – that hospitals could be swamped by AIDS cases. There, much effort went into collecting local epidemiological data in order to gather a picture of how the local epidemic was moving, leading in some cases to devising a care strategy to move the focus out of the hospital and into primary and community care settings.

Even without large numbers of patients, a small number of the localities studied showed a shrewd strategic grasp of HIV/AIDS from an early date (e.g. trying to check the seemingly remorseless build up of the acute sector by enhancing community care and preventive work). One or two could be seen as 'visionary' – the chance to do something new and exciting – but others in effect restated orthodox joint care planning models in a new field.

Most localities faced greater difficulties in the framing of policy. A lack of good quality epidemiological data was common, as was lack of information on the real workload being experienced in the various settings. In some cases there was an excessive focus on particular aspects of the problem (e.g. control of infection). Some were simply overwhelmed by the pace of change on the ground and an inability to implement agreed strategies, and a number of 'paper strategies' were encountered, which collapsed at the first hint of pressure. The ability to implement strategy therefore also depended on a consideration of the process of strategy implementation as well as generating a sound base in data and in policy.

A generalizable model?

We have attempted in this section to apply a model of features associated with receptivity to change, developed in a study of strategic service change within the NHS (Pettigrew et al. 1992), to a different change issue, HIV/ AIDS. Additionally we develop the model further by recognizing that there may be a temporal component to receptivity and ordering the features according to their significance at particular times in the chronological development of the issue. Hence, for this particular issue, 'environmental pressure' (stemming from the identification of HIV/AIDS and SMOs) came well before 'development of cooperative interorganizational networks'. A quite different ordering might be applicable to another change issue.

In general terms, we conclude that most of the original features of

receptivity for change were found to be present in our later study of HIV/
AIDS services, and that the inclusion of a temporal dimension in the model
adds to its explanatory power. This is an important finding as it begins to
suggest that there may be generic components to strategic change processes
in health care. We may also hypothesize that the model may be applicable
to processes of organizational change external to the NHS in organizations
in both the public and the private sector.

A look into the future – for management

Here we speculate more broadly about what the issues may be for
'management' (again very broadly defined) of HIV/AIDS services over the
next five or seven years. We assume that that this period will be marked
by a number of features very different from those found in our earlier
study of the response in the 1980s.

In particular, it appears that the period of crisis management has now
given way to the long haul. The epoch of rapid innovation and of charismatic leadership may be giving way to a period of consolidation, formalization and routinization. Moreover, unless another perceived crisis
supervenes, the political attention – and the level of special resourcing –
which has provided such an important umbrella in the past may be expected
to wane.

A continuing but changing epidemic

The epidemiological paradox is that HIV/AIDS may become less of an
issue but also more of a problem. The very basic point must be remembered that unlike many other health care issues, HIV is transmissible and
takes the form of an epidemic. While there is still much uncertainty, with
more epidemiological data available there does appear to be a better basis
for making medium-term forecasts about the incidence of new AIDS cases.

The latest epidemiological predictions (Public Health Laboratory Service
1993) suggest first of all a continuing modest upward growth in number
of new AIDS cases. The main change from the 1990 predictions is a
marked reduction in projected new cases among injecting drug users, and
whereas AIDS incidence in gay men may peak in 1993–94, the incidence
in those exposed heterosexually is expected to increase steadily, although
not exponentially. However, these predictions are subject to important
caveats. First, projections of a plateauing of cases among gay men will be
invalidated if indications of a recent increase in transmission rate are
confirmed. Second, the number of new cases due to heterosexual exposure
will be strongly influenced by the pattern of sexual relationships between
subsets of the population, about which little is currently known.

Assuming that the prediction of a steady, but not exponential increase in cases is borne out by events, there is unlikely to be any reigniting of a crisis mentality. On the other hand, the epidemic is unlikely to disappear, leaving behind expensive white elephants such as the tuberculosis sanitoria in the 1950s, and indeed, as Johnson (1992) points out, in the longer term we simply do not know what will happen:

> It is as erroneous to arrive at conclusions in the early 1990s about the eventual prevalence of HIV as it would have been to expect fifteenth century scientists in the decade after the introduction of syphilis to predict its devastating effect throughout Europe in subsequent centuries.

The most important trend may well be the growth in the number of heterosexual cases. At present, much of the service infrastructure has been built up in response to the needs of gay men, often through organizations run by them. The challenge is to ensure that the present facilities will be able to respond sympathetically to rising numbers of people with different needs, such as mothers with children. However, moving towards more generic forms of care may diminish the role of the pioneering SMOs, leading to a danger of loss of drive and energy and their, currently very important, voluntary contribution to service provision for those affected.

It is also important to note that planning service provision on the basis of predictions of numbers of cases of AIDS fails to take account of the considerable utilization of services by those with HIV infection who do not currently fulfil the criteria for an AIDS diagnosis. In one genitourinary medicine clinic we visited, less than a quarter of patients seen in the previous year had had AIDS, but the average number of clinic contacts per patient was eight, and 10 per cent had attended on between fifteen and twenty-seven occasions.

The quasi market and contracting

On the policy side, the main change over the next five years or so within health and social care is likely to be the further development of quasi markets and the purchaser/provider system. The NHS generally is reconfiguring into providers (NHS trusts) and purchasers (DHAs, GP fund holders) (Cm 555 1989). An even more radical change is apparent in social care (Cm 849 1989), where there is marked top-down pressure to increase the profile of voluntary and private providers.

HIV/AIDS services have, uniquely, not been included in the new contracting system up to this point, although in a sense HIV/AIDS services have operated according to 'contract-like' mechanisms ever since the birth of the special allocation, receiving a fixed sum of money and having to operate within that.

The relationship between those purchasing and providing services, the contract, has been defined in the NHS Review Working paper 2 (Cm 555 1989) as: 'to provide specified services in return for agreed funding'. This simple statement summarizes an extremely complex process. In order to contract effectively, access to current cost and caseload information is required, and judgements have to be made about the quality of provision and the future needs of different sectors of the population. In addition, decision-makers are expected to take into account the views of users, although the pace of development of the purchasing function is patchy and sometimes slow (Ferlie et al. 1993). Existing formal NHS information systems, as Bunch (1992) points out, frequently do not provide the detailed and varied data needed, while personnel with the skills needed in contracting are generally in short supply (Ham 1992). Setting and monitoring contracts is therefore a demanding task, even for discrete activities with quantifiable outcomes.

People with HIV/AIDS, however, require treatment and care involving a large number of different settings. Troop and Zimmern (1989) suggested that it was such groups of patients, requiring coordinated inputs from more than one source, that would provide the true test for the new arrangements:

> Contracts will also have to take into account the need for links between different parts of the service . . . at present many of these links are 'informal', based on close working relationships between different professional staff as much as on clearly defined organization. There are worries that with units and hospitals working to strict costings . . . much of this traditional coordination in health care between different services will be lost.

The complexity of collecting the data required to inform the development of contracting for HIV/AIDS services is perhaps at its greatest in some London health authorities, which carry a high caseload of HIV-infected people, many of whom are not local residents. However, even outside London, where prevalence is lower, the need to preserve confidentiality has hampered data collection. Bennett and Pettigrew (1991) found that monitoring and evaluation has in general been low on authorities' agendas. Tolley and Maynard (1990) noted particularly the lack of reliable outcome data, which increased the difficulty of monitoring expenditure.

In recognition of the problems likely to be involved in the implementation of contracting for HIV services, a joint NHS/Department of Health working party was set up in December 1990 to look at the feasibility of moving towards residence based funding. The working party concluded, in September 1992, that insufficient information was as yet available for a final decision on the implementation of contracting to be made, and that allocations of funds should continue to be made on a catchment basis. However, regions have been asked to continue to make progress in data collection and exchange in readiness for proposed change. It is likely that managing the transition to contracting will be a major task in the next few years.

New roles and responsibilities

The pattern of service development in the 1980s, we have argued, was shaped by clinical product champions, social movement organizations, and 'bureaucratic insurgents'. General managers played a generally reactive role, with some interesting and important exceptions. Public health played an important supportive and coordinating role, as conductor of the orchestra. These actors were innovating within governmental bureaux, and markets or 'quasi markets' were not significant features.

How might the cast of actors change in the 1990s? We suggest that three groups in particular are likely to play an increasingly important role. Taken together, they suggest a move away from Downsian processes of governmental innovation and towards more 'market-like' processes.

The first can be seen as the management of the increasingly large scale and perhaps deradicalized AIDS services organizations (Patton 1990). These organizations may develop as significant providers of service, led by professionalizing management. This fits with general trends observable in the voluntary sector (Butler and Wilson 1990) towards more active management, including the adoption of private sector models, concepts and even personnel. There are moves towards the 'rationalization' of organization design, and the emergence of a salariat skilled in conventional business-like management tasks and able to ensure that the organization survives in a new 'contract culture.' This move to more professionalized and business-like management may of course run counter to the strong cultural overlay of altruism and voluntarism, let alone the political motivation of many of those involved in SMOs.

Despite the history of failed attempts to draw clinicians into management from Griffiths onwards (DHSS 1983), an increasing number of hospitals, particularly NHS trusts, report the adoption of a clinical directorate structure, supported by new business manager posts (the language is significant). Education programmes have been laid on to help clinicians make the transition into management (Fitzgerald 1993).

Clinical directors, and their support staff, may well be much more market-like in their orientation, pressured by the NHS trust chief executives and boards of directors to demonstrate results. There may be an increasing emphasis on market research and on 'customer care initiatives.' There may even be some marketing activity, with better quality publications aimed at potential consumers.

A third new grouping will be the purchasers, especially purchasers addressing the needs of whole populations. At one level, the purchasers can also be seen as players in the quasi market, concerned to shop around to get the best bargain. Yet the value base of purchasing organizations should also be very different from those of the 'business-like' NHS trusts if they are to meet their proclaimed goal of acting as 'tribunes of the people'. As a result, there should be a concern within purchasing organizations to address issues of equity and meeting need, especially the needs of stigmatized groups. Their handling of the HIV/AIDS issue will prove a good test of their resolve. Concern has been expressed about the relatively slow pace of development of the needs assessment function which should lie at the heart of purchasing (Ferlie et al. 1993), but which too often has been overtaken by short-term contracting issues. On the other hand, HIV/AIDS might be seen as a promising test-bed for the development of the needs assessment function: its size makes it containable, and many of the clients are involved, middle class and articulate. It will be interesting to trace the development of needs assessment work in this area and to assess the impact of this work on the final purchasing plan for HIV/AIDS services.

The development of primary care

We are aware that in this book we have not been able to consider properly the role of primary care. This is partly because GP input was conspicuous by its absence in many of the localities studied. We suspect that the pattern may be changing, as some GPs build up interest and expertise, thus attracting referrals. There is also increasing pressure to move care out of the acute sector. It will be particularly interesting in the future to explore the role of GP fund holders, as purchasers of care, in this area.

Keeping the momentum going

A key theme is the question of how localities sustain the long-term development processes launched with such excitement in the mid-1980s. The sustaining of momentum is a theme of general significance for organizations, but one that has particular resonance in this field. We know that creating long-term change can be a difficult task, and that the institutionalization of apparently successful early innovations may be highly problematic. Goodman and Dean's 1982 study of organizations involved in major long-term change efforts, for instance, concluded: 'Our data painted a pessimistic picture. Change had been successfully introduced, some benefits had appeared but over time the majority of programs had become deinstitutionalized . . .'.

Are there any clues as to a possible way forward? One way of keeping a health issue to the forefront of management attention is for it to be a highly visible issue. Early in the epidemic key figures in the localities made much of opportunities to use the media and to give talks. Another mechanism was to publish articles and papers. Managers of HIV/AIDS services may increasingly need to cultivate media contacts and to be adept at spotting 'new angles' so as to generate a continuing flow of publicity for the issue.

There is also the question of building links between the services and local power figures, particularly with the management boards that are responsible for strategic direction. Many DHAs will discuss HIV/AIDS only once a year, when asked to endorse the annual AIDS Control Act return. It may be helpful to encourage a non-executive member to take a special interest in HIV/AIDS. In purchasing organizations, the Director of Public Health will nearly always be an executive director of the Authority, and thus play a key linking role to HIV/AIDS services.

Another aspect worth consideration in establishing and maintaining a high profile for HIV/AIDS is the number and status of those working in the field. Initially much activity was consultant-led, but such clinicians have progressively disengaged from managerial minutiae. Although AIDS Control Act returns show large numbers of people wholly or partly employed through the allocation, many are very junior or not visible. While localities now generally employ HIV/AIDS 'coordinators', they are frequently (especially in low prevalence areas) mainly associated with prevention activity, which, despite the rhetoric devoted to emphasizing its crucial importance, has traditionally been seen as of marginal significance. The status and remuneration of these posts is variable. However, some localities studied had recognized the need for high profile management posts as a focus for activity, signalling a greater importance accorded to the issue.

Development of interorganizational trust

The importance of informal relationships, and of the generation of trust, was highlighted in Chapter 7. The informal organization seemed more powerful than formal organizational arrangements in these areas of activity. Networks and small joint groups were highlighted as useful mechanisms.

This emphasizes the dangers that may emerge from any move to a highly 'arm's length' approach to contracting. In our view, quasi markets in health and social care should be seen as relational rather than neoclassical markets (Ferlie 1993). Dialogue and informal contacts between different purchasers and between purchasers and providers can be seen as an integral – and helpful – component to this kind of market.

Diffusion of learning to other services

We have argued that HIV/AIDS services have achieved – perhaps because of a conjunction of exceptional circumstances and exceptional people –

a high degree of user involvement, care coordination and provision of patient-sensitive services. There may well be lessons here for many other services which are trying to move in similar directions (e.g. oncology). Bentley and Adler (1990) thus suggest that HIV/AIDS can be seen as a model for the care of all patients with chronic conditions.

Yet we also found that there had been little learning about HIV/AIDS at a higher organizational level. Learning had taken place, but within relatively small compartments. A major managerial issue may be now to diffuse the learning that has taken place within HIV/AIDS settings to other settings through such devices as:

- Combining specialization and genericism: rotation of clinical and managerial staff through different settings.
- Use of educational and developmental opportunities to encourage reflection on what has been learned.
- Encouraging a more 'outward facing' relationship between HIV and other health care settings.

The encouragement of such learning can be seen as a legitimate focus for organizational development staff, where they exist at provider level. Sophisticated purchasers may also wish to address these issues in contract negotiation.

A look into the future – some rising theoretical themes

Alongside this changing managerial agenda for HIV/AIDS services may emerge some new organizational theoretical themes. Taking the lifecycle theory of public issues, many of the concepts utilized in this analysis of the response so far apparent reflect the early and fluid stages of the HIV/AIDS issue: clinical product champions, SMOs, crisis management and experiential learning.

We suspect that the HIV/AIDS issue will mature significantly in the 1990s as the pace of development slows. Innovators will give way to systems. Many of the significant investment decisions have already been made, even if only on a *de facto* basis, and will be difficult to shift. In these circumstances, the following themes may be of rising theoretical importance:

The characterization of social relations within quasi markets

We now see the progressive introduction of market-like arrangements throughout health and social care, and this trend is also likely to emerge within HIV/AIDS services. This in turn raises the key theoretical question of how we should conceive of quasi markets as a phenomenon. What might a quasi market look like in HIV/AIDS services?

We have considered elsewhere (Ferlie 1993) the relational view of markets at greater length. It was felt that the conventional view of an active marketeer, passive consumers and an atomistic market, restricted understanding of what actually happened in markets. The neoclassical model of markets assumed that markets are populated by individuals or by simple firms, yet economic life is often dominated by a small number of large and complex firms, which behave in a different way.

A number of important implications follow from seeing markets in more relational terms. Unlike individual consumers, corporate buyers might often interact with sellers. The relationship between organizations might display a complex history of adaptation, commitment, trust and conflict. Buyer–seller relationships are but one example of sets of relations that may shape a market, as buyer–buyer and seller–seller relations may also be important.

The interaction process is not seen as solely revolving around product–service exchange, but also includes important processes of social exchange, undertaken so as to reduce uncertainty and to build trust. The result may be a common value system, which emphasizes source loyalty. There is a tendency to 'keep things in the family', so that buyers – once locked into a set of relationships – may be relatively inert in seeking new sources of supply.

A relational market might well display the following 'signs and symptoms': (1) a relatively small number of well established buyers and sellers could be locked into long-run contracts or repeat buying; and (2) buying decisions are made on the basis of soft data (e.g. trust) as well as hard information. It may even be impossible to generate the hard information ideally required. The result is that 'reputation' is a key intangible asset on which providers trade. The market, in other words, is socially embedded (Granovetter 1985).

The impact of contracting on behaviour

Within quasi markets, management by contract replaces old-style management by hierarchy. So what are the long-term effects of the introduction of contracts on patterns of organizational and interorganizational behaviour? Will contracting erode traditional informal channels of communication, leading to an atomization of social relations?

This depends on the social properties of the contract as it evolves between purchaser and provider. Sociolegal scholars such as MacNeil (1974, 1978, 1983) (see also Hughes and Dingwall (1990) for an application of this approach to the study of contracting in health care) have distinguished between various types of contracts, commonly classical, neoclassical and relational.

The development of a 'relational' contract is seen as resulting from the increased duration and complexity of contracts. The contract becomes increasingly embedded in a social relation with its own history and norms.

Sociological purists might argue that the term 'relational contract' is almost a contradiction in terms, because in close relationships diffuse social norms of trust and reciprocity replace contracting as a means for restructuring recurring transactions. MacNeil (1983), however, contends that law facilitates the construction of relations because it fosters cooperation through internal and external values of contract behaviour based on many past contacts.

There is now the beginnings of an empirical literature on the effects of contracting on health and social care services generally. In particular, we should ask whether current changes such as the introduction of contracting are likely to accelerate or retard the future rate of innovation, particularly in the voluntary sector. According to the new thinking, much of the innovation apparent in the 1960s and 1970s in health and social care was 'provider-led.' The new arrangements are hence justified in the name of securing user led change, with purchasers acting as strong proxies. This is an ambitious agenda for new purchasing organizations to deliver and some fear that it is beyond their grasp. Common and Flynn's (1992) review of emergent forms of contracting between public purchasers and voluntary and private providers concluded:

> We fear however that the exercise (i.e. the purchaser provider split) will make Social Services more inward looking. The process of establishing the new market relationships between purchasers and providers may turn managers' and workers' attention away from the people who need the services. So far, contracting has led neither to neither increase in user choice or user control ...

In her review of current changes in the voluntary sector, Lewis (1993) specifically highlights the possible organizational effects of greater formalization and contract-driven relationships. She concluded that there was a danger of the erosion of more challenging developmental functions.

What can be said in the realm of theory about this question? Using the model suggested by Hage and Aiken (1967) and Hage and Dewar (1973), current trends contain a number of features that could be seen as retarding the rate of future innovation such as: a transfer of power from professionals to managers, rather than to users; increased formalization of contracts; greater stratification in the distribution of rewards; a high emphasis on volume production and an emphasis on efficiency and value for money.

Future work is needed to assess the extent to which these theoretical worries are or are not confirmed in data.

The study of interorganizational networks

Alongside markets and hierarchies as alternative devices for organizing social life stand 'networks' (Thompson 1991). These authors conceive of 'networks' as a flat organizational form, based on informal relationships between essentially equal social agents. They may be based on friendship, occupational grouping, gender or kin relationships. Networks themselves vary in strength, structure and shape.

We were struck by the importance of informal organizational processes in the development of HIV/AIDS services. Certainly interorganizational networks were found to be a key feature, often based on a strong common ideology, which crossed conventional organizational boundaries. This strong ideological base may be an unusual feature of networks in HIV/AIDS services. Often these networks were relatively restricted in size. Small-scale groupings forming around HIV/AIDS in the localities could be important arenas for the development of the interpersonal trust so necessary for collaboration. Where the actors involved in these networks possessed status and power, they could be an effective force for securing change. Where they did not, however, such networks could degenerate into 'talking shops.'

Whilst we are aware of the importance of these networks, we were not able to study them sufficiently in depth. How were they created and maintained? Do some of them in fact decay over time? Is there an actor who performs the role of a mobilizing focus for the network? Are some actors central to the network and others peripheral?

In conclusion

We hope in our analysis to have illuminated some of the organizational and management processes that shaped the development of HIV/AIDS services in the 1980s. This may superficially be seen as an unusual choice of topic for an organizational and managerial analysis, but we have argued that it illuminates a number of general organizational themes, such as the lifecycle approach to the study of public policy issues. Perhaps because of its containable size and associated social dramas, HIV/AIDS has proved to be a fascinating tracer issue. The challenge now is to carry this organizational analysis forward to what we would see as the latter stages of the issue lifecycle in the 1990s.

A second important contribution of this analysis has been to test some of our findings in relation to receptive and non-receptive contexts for change against a new and later set of data. It was interesting to note how many of the eight 'signs and symptoms' identified remained valid, providing some evidence that generic processes may be at work in shaping patterns of strategic change, at least in health care contexts. These are of course very early days, and more evidence is required before firm conclusions can be drawn. Nevertheless, we are heartened by the confirmatory evidence revealed in this study, which suggests that changes in health care may take generic rather than totally idiosyncratic forms.

References

ACMD (1982) *Treatment and Rehabilitation*. London: DHSS/HMSO.

Adler, M.W. (1988) Development of the epidemic, in *ABC of AIDS*. London: *British Medical Journal*.

Adler, M.W., Belsy, E.M., O'Connor, B.H., et al. (1978) Facilities and diagnostic criteria in sexually transmitted disease clinics in England and Wales, *British Journal of Venereal Diseases*, 54, 2–9.

Aggleton, P. and Homans, H. (eds) (1988) *Social Aspects of AIDS*. London: Falmer Press.

Alford, R. (1975) *Health Care Politics*. Chicago: University of Chicago Press.

Allen, M.P., Panian, S.K. and Lotz, R.E. (1979) Managerial succession and organisational performance: a recalcitrant problem revisited, *Administrative Science Quarterly*, 24, 167–80.

Annan, N. (1991) *Our Age: Portrait of a Generation*. London: Weidenfeld and Nicolson.

Argyris, C. and Schon, D.A. (1978) *Organisational Learning: A Theory in Action Perspective*. Reading, MA: Addison Wesley.

Arno, P. (1986) The non profit sector's response to the AIDS epidemic: community based services in San Francisco, *American Journal of Public Health*, 76(11), 1325–30.

Aron, R. (1977) *The Opium of the Intellectuals*. London: Greenwood.

Aves, G.M. (1969) *The Voluntary Worker in the Social Services*. London: Allen and Unwin.

Bandura, A. (1974) Behaviour theory and the models of man, *American Psychologist*, 29, 859–69.

Bartlett, F.C. (1932) *Remembering*. Cambridge: Cambridge University Press.

Bass, B.M. and Vaughan, J.A. (1966) *Training in Industry – The Management of Learning*. London: Tavistock Publications.

Beatty, R.P. and Zajac, E.J. (1987) CEO change and firm performance in large corporations: succession effects and manager effects, *Strategic Management Journal*, 8, 305–17.

Becher, T. (1989) *Academic Tribes and Territories*. Milton Keynes: Open University Press/Society for Research into Higher Education.

Becker, H.S. (1962) The nature of a profession, in *National Society for the Study of Education Sixty-First Year Book*. Chicago: University of Chicago Press.

Bennett, C.E. (1989) The Worcester Development Project: general practitioner satisfaction with a new community psychiatric service, *Journal of the Royal College of General Practitioners*, March, 106–9.

Bennett, C.E. (1993) DHPCs and collaborative working – issues for the future, in B. Evans, S. Sandberg and S. Watson (eds) *Healthy Alliances in HIV Prevention*. London: Health Education Authority.

Bennett, C.E. and Pettigrew, A.M. (1991) *Pioneering Services for Aids: The Response to HIV Infection in Four Health Authorities*. Final report of research for Department of Health, CCSC, University of Warwick.

Bennett, C.E., Ferlie, E.B. and Pettigrew, A.M. (1990) Developing services for HIV/ AIDS: organisational learning in *Department of Health Yearbook of Research and Development*. London: HMSO.

Bentley, C. and Adler, M.W. (1990) Choice cuts for patients with AIDS? *British Medical Journal*, 301, 15 Sept, 501–2.

Berger, P. and Luckmann, T. (1966) *The Social Construction of Reality*. Middlesex: Penguin Books.

Berridge, V. (1993) Introduction: AIDS and contemporary history, in V. Berridge and P. Strong (eds) *AIDS and Contemporary History*. Cambridge: Cambridge University Press.

Berridge, V. and Edwards, G. (1981) *Opium and the People*. London: Allen Lane.

Berridge, V. and Strong, P. (1992) AIDS policies in the United Kingdom, in E. Fee and D.M. Fox (eds) *AIDS: The Making of a Chronic Disease*. Oxford: University of California Press.

Berridge, V. and Strong, P. (1993) *AIDS and Contemporary History*. Cambridge: Cambridge University Press.

Beyer, J.M. (1981) Ideologies, values and decision making in organisations, in P.C. Nystrom and W.H. Starbuck (eds) *Handbook of organisational design*, vol 2. Oxford: Oxford University Press.

Blau, P. (1964) *Exchange and Power in Social Relations*. London: Wiley.

Booth, T.A. (1981) Collaboration between the health and social services: Part I, a case study of joint care planning, *Policy and Politics*, 9(1), 23–49.

Boudon, R. (1989) *The analysis of ideology*. Cambridge: Polity Press.

Brandt, A. (1988) AIDS in historical perspective: four lessons from the history of sexually transmitted diseases, *American Journal of Public Health*, 78(4), 369–92.

Brown, P. (ed.) (1989) *Perspectives in Medical Sociology*. California: Wadsworth Publishing Co. Inc.

Brown, J.S. and Duguid, P. (1991) Organisational learning and communities of practice: toward a unified view of working, learning and innovation, *Organisation Science*, 2(1), February, 40–57.

Bruner, J.S., Goodnow, J.J., and Austin, G.A. (1956) *A Study of Thinking*, New York: John Wiley.

Brunsson, N. (1982) The irrationality of action and action rationality: decisions, ideologies and organisational actions, *Journal of Management Studies*, 19(1), 29–44.

Bryder, L. (1990) The role of the MRC in science research policy. Paper given at the conference *AIDS and Contemporary History*, London School of Hygiene and Tropical Medicine, 5–6 April 1990.

Bucher, R. and Stelling, J. (1977) Characteristics of professional organisations, in R.L. Blankenship (ed.) *Colleagues in Organisations*. London: John Wiley (pp. 121–44).

Bucher, R. and Strauss, A. (1961) Professions in process, *American Journal of Sociology*, 66, 325–34.

Bunch, C. (1992) Developing a hospital information strategy: a clinician's view, *British Medical Journal*, 304, 1033–6.

Burgelman, R.A. and Sayles, L.R. (1986) *Inside Corporate Innovation: Strategy, Structure and Managerial Skills*. London: Collier Macmillan.

Burns, T. and Stalker, G.M. (1961) *The Management of Innovation*. London: Tavistock.

Butler, R. and Wilson, D. (1990) *Managing Voluntary and Non Profit Organisations*. London: Routledge.

Cangelosi, V.E. and Dill, W.R. (1965) Organisational learning: observations towards a theory, *Administrative Science Quarterly*, 10, 175–203.

Centers for Disease Control (1981) Pneumocystic pneumonia in homosexual men – Los Angeles, *Morbidity and Mortality Weekly Report*, 30, 250.

Challis, L., Fuller, S., Henwood, M., Klein, R., Plowden, W., Webb, A.L., Whittingham, P. and Wistow, G. (1988) *Joint Approaches to Social Policy*. Cambridge: Cambridge University Press.

Chandler, A.D. (1977) *The Visible Hand*. London: Harvard University Press.

Cherry, E.C. (1953) Some experiments on the recognition of speech, with one and with two ears, *Journal of Acoustic Sociology of America*, 25, 975–9.

Clark, B.R. (1972) The organisational saga in higher education, *Administrative Science Quarterly*, 17, 178–84.

Clift, S. and Stears, D. (1991) Moral perspectives and safer sex practice, in P. Aggleton, G. Hart and P. Davies (eds) *AIDS: Responses, Interventions and Care*. London: Falmer Press.

Cd 8189 (1916) *Royal Commission on Venereal Diseases: Final Report of the Commissioners*. London: HMSO.

Cmnd 247 (1957) *Report of the Committee on Homosexual Offences and Prostitution* (the Wolfenden Report). London: HMSO.

Cm 289 (1988) *Public Health in England: The Report of the Committee of Enquiry into the Future Development of the Public Health Function* (the Acheson Report). London: HMSO.

Cm 555 (1989) *Working for patients*. London: HMSO.

Cm 849 (1989) *Caring for people*. London: HMSO.

Cm 1523 (1991) *The health of the nation*. London: HMSO.

Cmnd 7615 (1979) *Report of the Royal Commission on the NHS*. London: HMSO.

Cohen, M.D. and March, J.G. (1974) *Leadership and Ambiguity: The American College President*. New York: McGraw-Hill.

Cohen, M.D., March, J.G. and Olsen, J.P. (1972) 'A garbage can model of organisational choice' *Administrative Science Quarterly*, 17(1), March, 1–25.
Common, R. and Flynn, N. (1992) *Contracting for Care*. York: Joseph Rowntree Foundation.
Connor, S. (1992) New dispute over royalties for HIV test, *British Medical Journal*, 304, 660.
Corbitt, G., Bailey, A.S. and Williams, G. (1990) HIV infection in Manchester, 1959, *The Lancet*, 336, 51.
Cranfield, S., Feinmann, C., Ferlie, E. and Walter, C. (1992) Managing service change in post HIV drugs services – a case study from Inner London, *British Journal of Addiction*, 87, 193–98.
Davenport-Hines, R. (1990) *Sex, Death and Punishment*. London: Collins.
David, M. (1984) Moral and material: the family in the right, in R. Levitas (ed.) *Ideology of the New Right*. Oxford: Polity Press.
Davies, B.P., Bebbington, A., Charnley, H., Baines, B., Ferlie, E., Hughes, M., and Twigg, J. (1990) *Resources, Needs and Outcomes in Community Based Care*. Aldershot: Avebury.
Department of Health (1988) *Report of the Working Group to Examine Workloads in GUM Medicine* (the Monks Report). London: Department of Health.
Dibble, V.K. (1962) Occupations and ideologies, *American Journal of Sociology*, 68, 229–41.
DHSS (1976) *Priorities for Health and Personal Social Services in England* (a Consultative Document). London: HMSO.
DHSS (1983a) *AIDS and How it Concerns Blood Donors*. London: HMSO.
DHSS (1983b) *NHS Management Enquiry Report* (the Griffiths Report). DA(83)38, London: DHSS.
DHSS (1988) *Short Term Prediction of HIV Infection and AIDS in England and Wales: Report of a Working Group* (the Cox Report). London: HMSO.
Downs, A. (1967) *Inside Bureaucracies*. Boston, MA: Little Brown.
Easton, G. and Rothschild, R. (1987) The influence of product and production flexibility on marketing strategy, in A.M. Pettigrew (ed.) *The Management of Strategic Change*. Oxford: Basil Blackwell.
Eckstein, H. (1960) *Pressure Group Politics: The Case of the British Medical Association*. London: Allen and Unwin.
Edwards, G. (1981) The Background, in G. Edwards and C. Busch (eds) *Drug Problems in Britain: A Review of Ten Years*. London: Academic Press.
Elliott, P. (1973) Professional ideology and social situation. *Sociological Review*, 21, 211–28.
Ferlie, E.B. (1992) The creation and evolution of quasi markets in the public sector: A problem for strategic management, *Strategic Management Journal*, 13, 79–97.
Ferlie, E.B. (1993) The NHS responds to HIV/AIDS, in P. Strong and V. Berridge (eds) *AIDS and Contemporary History*. Cambridge: Cambridge University Press.
Ferlie, E.B. and Bennett, C.E. (1992) Patterns of strategic change in health care: District Health Authorities respond to AIDS, *British Journal of Management*, 3, 21–37.
Ferlie, E.B. and Pettigrew, A.M. (1988) *The Management of Change in Paddington and North Kensington DHA: AIDS and Acute Sector Strategy*. Unpublished Case Study, Centre for Corporate Strategy and Change, University of Warwick.

Ferlie, E.B. and Pettigrew, A.M. (1990) Coping with Change in the NHS: A Frontline District's Response to AIDS, *Journal of Social Policy*, 19(2), 191–220.

Ferlie, E.B., Fitzgerald, L. and Ashburner, L. (1993) *The Challenge of Purchasing*. Research for Action Paper 7, Bristol: NHSTD.

Fitts P.M. and Posner, M.I. (1973) *Human performance*. London: Prentice/Hall International.

Fitzgerald, L. (1993) *Management Development for Consultants: Formative Evaluation of the Doctors in Business Schools Programme*. University of Warwick: CCSC.

Fitzsimons, D.W. (1993) 'Conference report: introduction, *AIDS Newsletter*, 8(10), 1–4.

Fox, D.M., Day, P. and Klein, R. (1989) The power of professionalism: policies for AIDS in Britain, Sweden, and the United States, *Daedalus*, 118(2), 93–112.

Freddi, G. (1989) Problems of organizational rationality in health systems: Political controls and policy options, in G. Freddi and J.W. Bjorkman (eds) *Controlling medical professionals: The comparative politics of health governance*. London: Sage.

Freeman, R. (1992) Governing the voluntary sector respose to AIDS: a comparative study of the UK and Germany, *Voluntas*, 3(1), 29–47.

Freidson, E. (1970) *Profession of Medicine: A Study of the Sociology of Applied Knowledge*. New York: Harper and Row.

Freidson, E. (1988) *Profession of Medicine: A Study of the Sociology of Applied Knowledge*, with a new Afterword. Chicago and London, University of Chicago Press.

French, J. and Adams, L. (1986) From analysis to synthesis, *Health Education Journal*, 45(2), 71–4.

Friend, J., Power, J. and Yewlett, L. (1974) *Public Planning: The Intercorporate Dimension*. London: Tavistock.

Gabbay, J. (1992) The health of the nation: seize the opportunity, *British Medical Journal*, 305, 129–30.

Geertz, C. (1973) *The Interpretation of Cultures*. New York: Basic Books.

de Geus, A.P. (1988) Planning as learning, *Harvard Business Review*, 66(2), 70–4.

Gladstone, F.J. (1979) *Voluntary action in a changing world*. London: Bedford Square Press.

Glaser, B.G. and Strauss, A.L. (1967) *The Discovery of Grounded Theory*. London: Weidenfeld and Nicolson.

Good, E. (1988) Individuals, interpersonal relations and trust, in D. Gambetta (ed.) *Trust*. Oxford: Basil Blackwell.

Goodman, P.S. and Dean, J.W. (1982) Creating long term organisational change, in P. Goodman, et al. *Change in Organisations*. London: Jossey Bass.

Granovetter, M.S. (1985) Economic action and social structure: The problem of embeddedness, *American Journal of Sociology*, 91(3), 481–510.

Hage, J. and Aiken, M. (1967) Program change and organisational properties, *American Journal of Sociology*, 72(5), 503–19.

Hage, J. and Dewar, R. (1973) Elite values (vs) organisational structure in predicting innovation, *Administrative Science Quarterly*, 18, 279–90.

Hall, O. (1949) Types of medical career, *American Journal of Sociology*, LV, 243–53.

Hall, S. and Jacques, M. (eds) (1983) *The Politics of Thatcherism*. London: Lawrence and Wishart.

Ham, C. (1992) More power to the purchaser, *British Medical Journal*, 304, 464.

Hardy, C. (1985) *Managing organisational closure*. London: Gower.

Harrigan, K.R. (1988) Joint ventures and competitive strategy, *Strategic Management Journal*, 9, 141–58.

Hebb, D.O. (1955) Drives and the CNS (conceptual nervous system), *Psychological Review*, 62, 243–54.

Hedberg, B.L.T. (1981) How organisations learn and unlearn, in P.C. Nystrom and W.H. Starbuck (eds) *Handbook of Organisational Design*, vol. 1. New York: Oxford University Press.

Hedberg, B.L.T., Nystrom, P.C. and Starbuck, W.H. (1976) Camping on see-saws: prescription for a self designing organisation, *Administrative Science Quarterly*, 21 March, 41–65.

Heraud, B. (1978) Professionalism and social work, unit 26, part 1, in *Social work, Community Work and Society* (course DE206). Buckingham: Open University Press.

Hermann, C.F. (1963) Some consequences of crisis which limit the visibility of organisations, *Administrative Science Quarterly*, 8(1), 61–82.

Hogwood, B.W. (1987) *From Crisis to Complacency?* Oxford: Oxford University Press.

Homans, H. and Aggleton, P. (1988) Health education, HIV infection and AIDS, in P. Aggleton and H. Homans (eds) *Social aspects of AIDS*. London: Falmer Press.

Huber, G.P. (1991) Organisational learning: The contributing processes and the literatures, *Organisation Science*, 2(1), 88–115.

Huczynski, A. and Buchanan, D. (1991) *Organisational Behaviour: An Introductory Text*, 2nd edn. London: Prentice-Hall International.

Hughes, D. and Dingwall, R. (1990) Sir Henry Maine, Joseph Stalin and the reorganisation of the National Health Service, *Journal of Social Welfare Law*, 5, 296–309.

Hull, C.L. (1943) *Principles of Behaviour*. New York: Appleton-Century-Crofts.

Hunter, D. (1980) *Coping with Uncertainty*. Chichester: Research Studies Press.

Janis, I.L. (1968) *Victims of Group Think: A psychological study of foreign policy decisions and fiascos*. Boston, MA: Houghton Mifflin.

Jelinek, M. and Schoonhoven, C.B. (1990) *Innovation Marathon*. Oxford: Basil Blackwell.

Jessop, B., Bonnett, K., Bromley, S. and Ling, T. (1984) Authoritarian populism, two nations and Thatcherism, *New Left Review*, 147, 32–60.

Jick, T.D. and Murray, V.V. (1982) The management of hard times: Budget cutbacks in public sector organisations, *Organisation Studies*, 3(2), 141–69.

Johnson, A.M. (1992) Home grown heterosexually acquired HIV infection, *British Medical Journal*, 304, 1125–6.

Johnson, G. (1990) Managing strategic change – the role of symbolic action, *British Journal of Management*, 1(4), 183–200.

Johnson, G. and Scholes, K. (1984) *Exploring Corporate Strategy*. London: Prentice-Hall International.

Johnston, A.V. (1975) Revolution by involvement, *Accountancy Age*, 7(36), 17.

Jones, A.M. and Hendry, C. (1992) *The Learning Organisation: A Review of Literature and Practice*. London: Human Resource Management Partnership.

Kelly, G. (1955) *The Psychology of Personal Constructs*, vols 1 and 2. New York: Norton.

de Kervasdoue, J. (1981) Institutions, organisations, medical disciplines and the dissemination of research results, *Organisation Studies*, 2(3), 246–66.

Kimberly, J., Miles, R., and associates (1980) *The Organisational Life Cycle*. San Francisco: Jossey Bass.

Kingsley, S. (1981) Voluntary action: innovation and experiment as criteria for funding, *Home Office Research Unit Bulletin*, 11, 7–10.

Kinston, W. (1983) Hospital organisation and structure and its effect on inter-professional behaviour and the delivery of care, *Social Science of Medicine*, 17(16), 1159–70.

Klandermans, B. (1992) The social construction of protest and multi-organisational fields, in A.D. Morris and C. McClurg Mueller (eds) *Frontiers in Social Movement Theory*. New Haven, CT and London: Yale University Press.

Kleiman, P. (1989) *Lessons for the Future: Report of an Evaluation Study of the Manchester AIDS in Education Group*. Manchester: CRISAH, University of Manchester.

Kogut, B. (1988) Joint ventures: theoretical and empirical perspectives, *Strategic Management Journal*, 9, 319–32.

Lawrence, P.R. and Lorsch, J.W. (1967) *Organisation and Environment*. Cambridge, MA: Harvard Graduate School of Business Administration.

Levine, S. and White, P. (1961) Exchange as a conceptual framework for the study of interorganisational relationships, *Administrative Science Quarterly*, 5, 583–601.

Levine, C.H., Rubin, I.S., and Wolohojian, G.G. (1982) Managing organisational retrenchment, *Administration and Society*, 14(1), 101–36.

Lewis, J. (1993) Developing the mixed economy of care: emerging issues for voluntary organizations, *Journal of Social Policy*, 22(2), 173–92.

Local Authority Association (Officer Working Group On Aids) (1988) *HIV infection and drug use*. London: Association of Metropolitan Authorities.

Lofland, J. (1971) *Analysing Social Settings*. Belmont, CA: Wadsworth.

Lohdahl, T.M. and Mitchell, S.M. (1980) Drift in the development of innovative organisations, in J.R. Kimberly, R.H. Miles et al. (eds) *The Organisational Life Cycle*. San Francisco: Jossey Bass.

Lussier, R. (1984) The history of health education, in L. Robinson and W. Alles (eds) *Health Education: Foundations for the Future*. Philadelphia, PA: Mosby.

Lyles, M.A. (1981) Formulating strategic problems: empirical analysis and model development, *Strategic Management Journal*, 2, 61–75.

Lyles, M.A. (1990) A research agenda for strategic management in the 1990s, *Journal of Management Studies*, 27, 363–75.

McCarthy, J.D and Wolfson, M. (1992) Consensus movements, conflict movements, and the cooptation of civic and state infrastructures, in A.D. Morris and C. McClurg Mueller (eds) *Frontiers in Social Movement Theory*. New Haven, CT and London: Yale University Press.

Maccoby, E.E. (1959) Role-taking in childhood and its consequences for social learning, *Child Development*, 30, 239–52.

Macneil, I. (1974) The many futures of contracts, *Southern California Law Review*, 47, 691–816.

Macneil, I. (1978) Contracts: adjustments of long term economic relations under conditions of classical, neo classical and relational contract law, *Northwestern University Law Review*, 72, 854–906.

Macneil, I. (1983) Values in contract: internal and external, *Northwestern University Law Review*, 77, 340.

Mann, J.M. and Carballo, M. (1989) Social cultural and political aspects: overview, *AIDS 1989: 3 (suppl. 1)*: S221–S223.

March, J.G. (1988) *Decisions and Organisations*. Oxford: Basil Blackwell.

March, J.G. (1992) *The evolution of evolution*. Paper presented to the *Conference of Evolutionary Dynamics of Organisations*, New York University, 10–12 January 1992.

March, J.G. and Olsen, J.P. (1976) *Ambiguity and Choice in Organisations*. Bergen: Universitetsforlaget.

Meyer, A.D. (1982) Adapting to environmental jolts, *Administrative Science Quarterly*, 27, 515–37.

Miller, D. and Friesen, P.M. (1982) The longitudinal analysis of organisations: A methodological perspective, *Management Science*, 28(9), 1013–34.

Minsky, M. (1977) Frame-system theory, in P.N. Johnson Laird and P.C. Wason (eds) *Thinking: Readings in Cognitive Science*. Cambridge: Cambridge University Press.

Ministry of Health (1926) *Report of the Departmental Committee on Morphine and Heroin Addiction*. London: HMSO.

Mintzberg, H. (1989) *Mintzberg on Management*. New York: The Free Press.

Mishler, E.G. (1981) Critical perspectives on the bio-medical model, in E.G. Mishler, et al. (eds) *Social Contexts of Health, Illness and Patient Care*. Cambridge: Cambridge University Press.

Morgan, G. (1986) *Images of organisation*. London: Sage.

Morris, A.D. (1992) Political consciousness and collective action, in A.D. Morris and C. McClurg Mueller (eds) *Frontiers in Social Movement Theory*. New Haven, CT and London: Yale University Press.

Moss Kanter, R. (1972) *Commitment and Community in Communes and Utopias in Sociological Perspective*. Cambridge, MA: Harvard University Press.

Moss Kanter, R. (1989) *When Giants Learn to Dance*. London: Unwin.

Mowrer, O.H. (1950) *Learning Theory and Personality Dynamics*. New York: Ronald Press.

Muraskin, W. (1993) Hepatitis B as a model (and anti-model) for AIDS, in V. Berridge and P. Strong (eds) *AIDS and Contemporary History*. Cambridge: Cambridge University Press.

Nadler, D.A. (1983) *Concepts for the Management of Organisational Change*. Delta Consulting Group.

Nadler, D.A. and Tushman, M. (1990) Beyond the charismatic leader: leadership and organisational change, *California Management Review*, 32(2), 77–97.

National Audit Office (1991) *HIV and AIDS Related Health Services*. Report by the Comptroller and Auditor General. London: HMSO.

Normann, R. (1985) Developing capabilities for organisational learning, in J.M. Pennings et al. (eds) *Organisational Strategy and Change*. London: Jossey Bass.

Ottaway, R.N. (1976) A change strategy to implement new norms, new styles and new environment in the work organisation, *Personnel Review*, 5(1), 13–18.

Padgug, R.A. and Oppenheimer, G.M. (1992) Riding the tiger: AIDS and the gay community, in E. Fee and D.M. Fox (eds) *AIDS: The Making of a Chronic Disease*. Oxford: University of California Press.

Parsons, T. (1951) *The social system*. New York: The Free Press.

Patton, C. (1990) *Inventing AIDS*. London: Routledge.

Pearson, G. (1978) Welfare on the move, unit 4, in 'Social Work, Community Work and Society' (Course DE206). Buckingham: Open University Press.

Pedler, M., Boydell, T. and Burgoyne, J. (1988) *Learning Company Project: A Report on Work Undertaken October 1987 – April 1988*. Unpublished document, University of Lancaster.

Perrow, C. and Guillen, M. (1990) *The AIDS Disaster*. New Haven, CT and London: Yale University Press.

Peters, T. and Waterman, R.H. (1982) *In Search of Excellence*. London: Harper and Row.

Pettigrew, A.M. (1973) *The Politics of Organisational Decision Making*. London: Tavistock.

Pettigrew, A.M (1975) Strategic aspects of the management of specialist activity, *Personnel Review*, 4, 5–13.

Pettigrew, A.M. (1979) On studying organisational cultures, *Administrative Science Quarterly*, 24, 570–81.

Pettigrew, A.M. (1985) *The Awakening Giant*. Oxford: Basil Blackwell.

Pettigrew, A.M. (1990) Longitudinal field research on change: theory and practice, *Organisation Science*, 3(1), 267–92.

Pettigrew, A.M. and Whipp, R. (1991) *Managing Change for Competitive Success*. Oxford: Basil Blackwell.

Pettigrew, A.M., McKee, L. and Ferlie, E.B. (1988) Understanding change in the NHS, *Public Administration*, 66(3), 297–317.

Pettigrew, A.M., Ferlie, E.B. and McKee, L. (1992) *Shaping Strategic Change: Making Change in Large Organisations – the Case of the NHS*. London: Sage.

Peutherer, J.F., Edmond, E., Simmonds, P., Dickson, J.D. and Bath, G.E. (1985) HTLV-III antibody in Edinburgh drug addicts, *The Lancet*, November 16, 1129.

Pfeffer, J. and Salancik, G.R. (1978) *The External Control of Organisations: A Resource Dependence Perspective*. New York: Harper and Row.

Philips, J. (1988) Coming to terms, in B. Cant and S. Hemmings (eds) *Radical Records: Thirty Years of Lesbian and Gay History, 1957–1987*. London: Routledge.

Pollitt, C. (1990) *Managerialism and the Public Services*. Oxford: Basil Blackwell.

Public Health Laboratory Service (1990) *Acquired Immune Deficiency Syndrome in England and Wales to end 1993: projections using data to end September 1989*. Communicable Disease Report (the Day Report). London: HMSO.

Public Health Laboratory Service (1993) *The incidence and prevalence of AIDS and other severe HIV disease in England and Wales for 1992–1997: projections using data to the end of June 1992*. Communicable Disease Report (the Day Report), 3 (suppl. 1), S1–17. London: HMSO.

Pye, M., Kapila, M., Buckley, G. and Cunningham, D. (eds) (1989) *Responding to the AIDS challenge: A comparative study of local AIDS programmes in the United Kingdom*. Harlow: Health Education Authority/Longman.

Rhodes, R.A.W. (1988) *Beyond Westminster and Whitehall*. London: Unwin Hyman.

Robertson, J.R., Bucknall, A.B.V., Welsby, P.D., Roberts, J.J.K., Inglis, J.M., Peutherer, J.F. and Brettle, R.P. (1986) Epidemic of AIDS related Virus (HTLV-III/LAV) infection amongst intravenous drug abusers, *British Medical Journal*, 292, 527.

Roe, A. (1952) A psychologist examines sixty-four eminent scientists, *Scientific American*, 187, 21–5.

Rooff, M. (1957) *Voluntary Societies and Social Policy*. London: Routledge and Kegan Paul.

Rothwell, R. (1976) Intracorporate entrepreneurs, *Management Decision*, 13(3), 142–54.

Rothwell, R. and Zegweld, W. (1982) *Innovation and the Small and Medium Sized Firm*. London: Frances Pinter.

Sainsbury, E. (1977) *The Personal Social Services*. London: Pitman

Sapolsky, H.M. and Boswell, S.L. (1992) The history of transfusion AIDS, in E. Fee and D.M. Fox (eds) *AIDS: The Making of a Chronic Disease*. Oxford: University of California Press.

Sarason, S. (1976) *The Creation of Settings and the Future Societies*. San Francisco: Jossey Bass.

Schein, E.H. (1985) *Organisational Culture and Leadership*. San Francisco: Jossey Bass.

Schramm-Evans, Z. (1990) Responses to AIDS: 1986–1987, in P. Aggleton, P. Davies, and G. Hart (eds) *AIDS: Individual, Cultural and Policy Dimensions*. London: Falmer Press.

Scruton, R. (1986) *Sexual Desire*. London: Weidenfeld and Nicolson.

Seebohm, F. (1968) *Report of the Committee on Local Authority and Allied Personal Social Services*. London: HMSO.

Seliger, M. (1976) *Ideology and Politics*. London: Allen and Unwin.

Shils, E. (1968) Ideology, *International Encyclopaedia of the Social Sciences*, 7, 66–76.

Shilts, R. (1987) *And the Band Played On*. Middlesex: Penguin.

SHHD (1986) *HIV Infection in Scotland. Report of the Scottish Committee on HIV infection and intravenous drug misuse* (the McClelland Report). London: HMSO.

Sim, A.J.W. and Dudley, H.A.F. (1988) Surgeons and HIV, *British Medical Journal*, 296, 9.

Simon, H.A. (1953) Birth of an organisation: the economic cooperation administration, *Public Administration Review*, 13, 236.

Singh, J.V., House, D.J. and Tucker, D.J. (1986) Organisational change and organisational mortality, *Administrative Science Quarterly*, 31, 587–611.

Skinner, B.F. (1953) *Science and Human Behaviour*. New York: Macmillan.

Snow, D.A. and Benford, R.D. (1992) Master frames and cycles of protest, in A.D. Morris and C. McClurg Mueller (eds) *Frontiers in Social Movement Theory*. New Haven, CT and London: Yale University Press.

Social Services Select Committee (1987) *Problems associated with AIDS*, Session 1986–87, 3rd Report HCP 182. London: House of Commons.

Soeters, J.L. (1986) Excellent companies as social movements, *Journal of Management Studies*, 23(3), 299–312.

Sontag, S. (1988) *AIDS and its Metaphors*. Middlesex: Penguin.

Stacey, M. (1988) *The Sociology of Health and Healing*. London: Unwin and Hyman.

Starbuck, W.H. (1982) Congealing oil: Inventing ideologies to justify acting ideologies out, *Journal of Management Studies*, 19(1), 3–27.

Starbuck, W.H., Greve, A. and Hedberg, B.L.T. (1978) Responding to crisis, *Journal of Business Administration*, 9, 111–37.

Stimson, G.V., Aldritt, L.J., Dolan, K.A., Donoghoe, M.C. and Lart, R.A. (1988) *Injecting Equipment Schemes: Final Report, November 1988*. London: Monitoring Research Group, Goldsmiths College.

Stockford, D. (1992) Developments in purchasing and contracting, in B. Evans, S. Sandberg and S. Watson (eds) *Healthy Alliances in HIV Prevention*. London: Health Education Authority.

Stocking, B. (1985) *Initiative and Inertia in the NHS*. London: Nuffield Provincial Hospitals Trust.

Street, J. (1993) A fall in interest? British AIDS policy, 1986–1990, in V. Berridge and P. Strong (eds) *AIDS and Contemporary History*. Cambridge: Cambridge University Press.

Strong, P. (1990) Epidemic psychology: a model, *Sociology of Health and Illness*, 12 no. 3, 249–59.

Strong, P. and Berridge, V. (1990) No one knew anything: some issues in British AIDS Policy, in P. Aggleton, P. Davies and G. Hart (eds) *AIDS: Individual, Cultural and Policy Dimensions*. London: Falmer Press.

Strong, P. and Robinson, J. (1990) *The NHS under New Management*. Buckingham: Open University Press.

Szasz, T. (1975) *Ceremonial Chemistry: The Ritual Persecution of Drugs, Addicts and Pushers*. London: Routledge and Kegan Paul.

Tarrow, S. (1983) *Struggling to Reform: Social Movements and Policy Change during Cycles of Protest*. Ithaca, NY: Western Societies Program, Cornell University.

Thomas, E.H. and Fox, D.M. (1989) AIDS on Long Island – the regional history of an epidemic, 1981–86, *Long Island Historical Journal*, 1(2), 93–111.

Thompson, J. (1984) *Studies in the Theory of Ideology*. Cambridge: Polity Press.

Thompson, G. (1991) Networks: introduction, in G. Thompson, J. Frances, R. Levacic and J. Mitchell (eds) *Markets, Hierarchies and Networks: The Co-ordination of Social Life*. London: Sage (pp. 243–345).

Tolley, K. and Maynard, A. (1990) *Government funding of HIV/AIDS medical and social care*. Discussion Paper 70, University of York Centre for Health Economics, Health Economics Consortium.

Tolman, E.C. (1932) *Purposive Behaviour in Animals and Men*. New York: Appleton-Century-Crofts.

Toren, M. (1969) Semi professionalism and social work: a theoretical perspective, in A. Etzioni (ed) *The Semi-professions and their Organisation*. New York: The Free Press.

Touraine, A. (1981) *The Voice and the Eye: An Analysis of Social Movements*. Cambridge: Cambridge University Press.

Troop, P. and Zimmern, R. (1989) *A Model for the Post-White Paper NHS*. NHS Management Bulletin, NHS Management Executive.

Turner, B.A. (1976) The organisational and interorganisational development of disasters, *Administrative Science Quarterly*, 21, 378–97.

Turner, V.W. (1957) *Schizm and Continuity in an African Society*. Manchester: Manchester University Press.

Tyhurst, J.S. (1951) Individual reactions to community disaster: The natural history of psychiatric phenomena, *American Journal of Psychiatry*, 107, 764–9.

Wallis, R. (1976) Moral indignation and the media: an analysis of the NVLA. *Sociology*, 10(2), 271–95.

Watney, S. (1988) Visual AIDS: advertising ignorance, in P. Aggleton and H. Homans (eds) *Social Aspects of AIDS*. London: Falmer Press.

Webb, A. (1991) Coordination: a problem in public sector management, *Policy and Politics*, 19(4), 229–41.

Weeks, J. (1989) AIDS: the intellectual agenda, in P. Aggleton, P. Davies and G. Hart (eds) *AIDS: Social Representations, Social Practices*. Lewes: Falmer Press.

Welsh, J.A. and White, J.F. (1981) Converging on the characteristics of entrepreneurs, in K.H. Vesper (ed.) *Frontiers of Entrepreneurship Research 1981*. Proceedings of the 1981 Babson College Entrepreneurship Research Conference. Wellesley, MA: Centre for Entrepreneurial Studies, Babson College.

Wilensky, H.L. (1964) The professionalisation of everyone? *American Journal of Sociology*, 70(2), 137–58.

Wilson. B, (ed.) (1967) *Patterns of Sectarianism*. London: Heinemann.

Wilson, D. (1992) The strategic challenges of co-operation and competition in British voluntary organisations: towards the next century, *Non Profit Management and Leadership*, 2(3), 239–54.

Wolfenden Committee (1977) *The Future of Voluntary Organisations*. London: Croom Helm.

Yin, R.K. (1989) *Case Study Research: Design and Methods*. Beverley Hills, CA: Sage.

Zald, M.N. and Berger, M.A. (1978) Social movements in organisations: coup d'etat, insurgency and mass movements, *American Journal of Sociology*, 83(4), 823–61.

Index

PRIVATIZATION AND REGULATORY CHANGE IN EUROPE

Michael Moran and Tony Prosser (eds)

Privatization and deregulation have been dominant symbols in economic policy across Europe in recent years. How far has the reality matched these symbols? Are we living in an era when the market is triumphant at the expense of state control of economic life? This book examines the analytical debates and the experience of a wide range of European countries, both east and west, including contributions from both lawyers and political scientists. Studies of the present state of privatization in the former Communist economies are matched by surveys of the state of deregulation in some of the most important capitalist states of western Europe. The authors emphasize the extent to which economic change is shaped by political strategies and interests, and the extent to which economic change has wide ranging constitutional implications.

This book will be essential reading for all those interested in making sense of the revolutionary changes now sweeping over the economies of the industrial world.

Contents
Introduction: politics, privatization and constitutions – Regulatory reform and privatization in Germany – Privatization and regulatory change: the case of Great Britain – Deregulation and privatization in Italy – Privatization and regulatory change: the case of Czechoslovakia – Privatization and regulatory change: the case of Poland – Environmental policy and regulatory change in Hungary – The political economy of ecological modernization: creating a regulated market for environmental quality – Conclusion: from national uniqueness to supra-national constitution – Index.

Contributors
Sabino Cassese, Michal du Vall, Kenneth Hanf, Jeremy Leaman, Tadeusz Markowski, Michael Mejstrik, Michael Moran, Istvan Pogany, Tony Prosser, Milan Sojka.

176pp   0 335 19072 3 (Paperback)   0 335 19073 1 (Hardback)

WHATEVER HAPPENED TO LOCAL GOVERNMENT?

Allan Cochrane

In the 1980s British local government was at the eye of the political storm. Councils were blamed for overspending and central government was blamed for threatening to bring an end to local democracy. In 1990 a new local tax – the poll tax – proved so unpopular that it helped to bring an end to Margaret Thatcher's reign as Prime Minister. But what has really happened to local government over the last fifteen years? What do the changes tell us about the nature of British politics in the 1990s? And what do they mean for the future direction of local government?

These questions are at the heart of this book, which argues that it is necessary fundamentally to reappraise the ways in which we understand local government. Allan Cochrane develops a wide ranging argument, drawing on material from across the traditional divisions created by academic disciplines and theoretical systems to show that local government in Britain will never be the same again. It needs to be seen as just one element in a more complex local welfare state, which is itself being transformed to fit in with a new (business-led) agenda for welfare.

Contents

160pp   0 335 19011 1 (Paperback)

IMPLEMENTING HOUSING POLICY

Peter Malpass and Robin Means (eds)

Following its radical housing policy reforms of the early 1980s the British government carried out a fundamental policy review in 1986–87 and launched into a
further bout of major legislative change in the Housing Act 1988, and the Local
Government and Housing Act 1989. These Acts introduced a range of new policy
instruments which are being applied with differing degrees of success. *Implementing
Housing Policy* provides the first full and detailed account of the new housing
policy in action, each chapter written by a well-known specialist in the field.

But the book is much more than a policy review; its distinctive focus on implementation makes it a particularly valuable addition to the literature. Implementation too often remains a taken-for-granted aspect of the policy process, but the
contributors to this book explicitly address the importance and complexity of
the policy-action relationship. As a result the book will appeal to a wide range
of readers interested in public policy and policy processes in general.

Contents
*Introduction: focus and outline – Perspectives on implementation – Housing policy
and the housing system since 1979 – The re-privatization of housing associations
– Rebuilding the private rented sector? – Remodelling a HAT: the implementation
of the Housing Action Trust legislation 1987–92 – The new financial regime for
local authority housing – Housing renewal in an era of mass home ownership –
The enabling role for local housing authorities: a preliminary evaluation – The
decentralization of housing services – Large-scale voluntary transfers – The politics
of implementation – Index.*

Contributors
Glen Bramley, Ian Cole, Valerie Karn, Peter Kemp, Philip Leather, Sheila Mac-
kintosh, Peter Malpass, Robin Means, David Mullins, Pat Niner, Bill Randolph,
Moyra Riseborough, Matthew Warburton.

208pp   0 335 15750 5 (Paperback)   0 335 15751 2 (Hardback)